Death Defiers Editorial Staff

Managing Editor: **Jack Croft**

Senior Editor: **Stephen C. George**

Writers: **Selene Yeager, Kelly Garrett, Kenneth Winston Caine, Perry Garfinkel, Brian Paul Kaufman**

Contributing Writers: **Jennifer A. Barefoot, Carol J. Gilmore, Jennifer L. Kaas, Mary S. Mesaros, Deanna Moyer, Deborah Pedron, Lorna S. Sapp**

Assistant Research Manager: **Jane Unger Hahn**

Lead Researcher: **Deanna Moyer**

Editorial Researchers: **Jennifer A. Barefoot, Christine Dreisbach, Jan Eickmeier, Carol J. Gilmore, Jennifer L. Kaas, Mary Kittel, Mary S. Mesaros, Kathryn Piff, Lorna S. Sapp, Lucille Uhlman, Nancy Zelko**

Copy Editor: **David R. Umla**

Associate Art Director: **Charles Beasley**

Cover Designer and Series Art Director: **Tanja Lipinski-Cole**

Series Designer: **John Herr**

Cover Photographer: **Mitch Mandel**

Part Opener Illustrator: **Bryon Thompson**

Chapter Opener Illustrator: **Alan Baseden**

Layout Designer: **Donna G. Rossi**

Manufacturing Coordinator: **Melinda B. Rizzo**

Office Manager: **Roberta Mulliner**

Office Staff: **Julie Kehs, Mary Lou Stephen**

Rodale Health and Fitness Books

Vice President and Editorial Director: **Debora T. Yost**

Executive Editor: **Neil Wertheimer**

Design and Production Director: **Michael Ward**

Research Manager: **Ann Gossy Yermish**

Copy Manager: **Lisa D. Andruscavage**

Production Manager: **Robert V. Anderson Jr.**

Studio Manager: **Leslie M. Keefe**

Associate Studio Manager: **Thomas P. Aczel**

Book Manufacturing Director: **Helen Clogston**

Photo Credits

Page 146: **Courtesy of Robert Mondavi Vineyards**

Page 148: **Darren Carroll**

Page 150: **Courtesy of BEFIT Enterprises**

Page 152: **Robert Clark**

Page 162: **Corbis-Bettmann**

Page 163: **Everett Collection**

Page 164: **National League of Baseball**

Page 165: **Corbis-Bettmann**

Back flap: **Culver Pictures**

Contents

Newca:

To be r

1

18 (

1

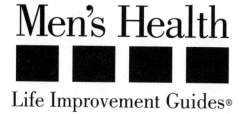

Men's Health

Life Improvement Guides®

Death Defiers

Beat the Men-Killers
and Live Life to the Max

By Selene Yeager, Kelly Garrett,
and the Editors of Men'sHealth Books

Rodale Press, Inc.
Emmaus, Pennsylvania

Notice

This book is intended as a reference volume only, not as a medical manual. The information given here is designed to help you make informed decisions about your health. It is not intended as a substitute for any treatment that may have been prescribed by your doctor. If you suspect that you have a medical problem, we urge you to seek competent medical help.

Other titles in the *Men's Health Life Improvement Guides* series:

Command Respect	*Good Loving*	*Sex Secrets*	*Symptom Solver*
Fight Fat	*Maximum Style*	*Stress Blasters*	*Vitamin Vitality*
Food Smart	*Powerfully Fit*	*Stronger Faster*	

Library of Congress Cataloging-in-Publication Data

Yeager, Selene.
　　Death defiers : beat the men-killers and live life to the max / by
Selene Yeager, Kelly Garrett, and the editors of Men's Health Books.
　　　　p.　　cm. — (Men's health life improvement guides)
　　Includes index.
　　ISBN 1–57954–088–0　hardcover
　　ISBN 0–87596–476–1　paperback
　　1. Men—Health and hygiene.　2. Longevity.　I. Garrett, Kelly.
II. Men's Health Books.　III. Title.　IV. Series.
RA777.8.Y43　1998
613'.04234—dc21
　　　　　　　　　　　　　　　　　　　　　　98–14392

Distributed in the book trade by St. Martin's Press

2　4　6　8　10　9　7　5　3　1　　hardcover
2　4　6　8　10　9　7　5　3　1　　paperback

— OUR PURPOSE —

"*We inspire and enable people to improve their lives and the world around them.*"

Part Five

Real-Life Scenarios

Quest for the Best

You Can Do It!

Introduction

You Wanna Live Forever?

If you go to the movies, you know what Hollywood considers to be the leading men-killers. Femmes fatales with ice water in their veins and an ice pick under the bed. Towering infernos that not even Fred Astaire can dance away from. Earthquakes that shake Los Angeles harder than the Laker Girls. Volcanos that spew rivers of molten lava. Mammoth sharks. Prehistoric dinosaurs. Arnold Schwarzenegger's Terminator.

While those sensational plot lines may top the box-office lists, it probably won't surprise you to learn that none of them top the list of the leading causes of death among American men. No, the real reasons that men die before their time have far less box-office potential than drop-dead gorgeous blondes or marauding cyborgs. But your odds of escaping the real-life men-killers are much better than outrunning a rampaging *Tyrannosaurus rex* or outswimming a great white shark. That's because men, in a very real sense, control their own destinies when it comes to health.

It's estimated that genetics is roughly 20 percent responsible for how long we live. The rest is up to us. The statistics bear that out. The number one killer of men is heart disease. Number two is cancer. Those two causes account for more than twice as many deaths as the next eight men-killers *combined*, according to the National Center for Health Statistics. And that's just the tip of a Top 10 list that includes accidents, lung disease, suicide, and murder, most of which have little or nothing to do with genetics, so much as they have to do with the life choices we make.

To be sure, men don't always make the best decisions in this arena. One of the saddest commentaries I've ever heard on the state of men's health came from my boyhood idol, Mickey Mantle (whose cautionary tale you'll find in these pages). Toward the end, the Mick said: "If I knew I was going to make it to 50, I would have taken better care of myself."

With *Death Defiers*, you need never utter those words.

Here, you'll find everything you need to lead you away from the long downhill road to physical and mental decline. We'll show you how to make the difference between dying before your time and living beyond your years. And again, it takes just a few choices, wisely made. What to eat. How to exercise. How to handle stress. When to play it safe. When to treat yourself. And when to ask for help.

We did not intend *Death Defiers* to be a handbook for the cautious, oh no. That's why you'll also discover the ingredients to living a life that's full and rich. Inside, you'll meet men who've made it to their 100th birthday by virtue of attitude and good humor. You'll discover that you won't have to sacrifice any of your favorite things in life in order to get more out of it. (In fact, some of the best things in life—hot sex, a good drink, a warm bed—can actually help you live longer and better.) And if you want to know what it takes to be immortal, we have a whole menu of ways you can extend your influence far beyond the span of any human lifetime.

Hmmm. An ordinary man uncovers the secret to cheating death and living forever. Sounds like a movie plot, you say? Not at all. This is real life.

This is *your* life.

Jack Croft

Jack Croft
Managing Editor, *Men's Health* Books

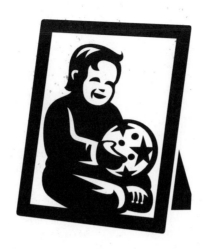

Part One

Live Long and Prosper

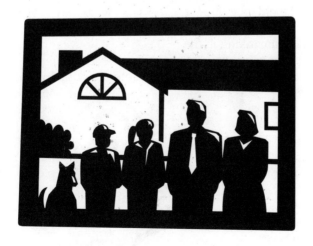

Why We Die

It's a Small World after All

Men in white lab coats have been pondering the reasons behind our imminent mortality as long as there have been men to wear white coats. And, anticlimactic though it may seem, they say that sex is the answer. We reproduce. We age. And we die.

"The price we pay for sex is death," explains S. Jay Olshansky, Ph.D., associate professor, biodemographer, and scientist in the department of medicine at the University of Chicago, Division of Biological Sciences, Pritzker School of Medicine. Once we have reproduced and passed on our genes, we as individuals are disposable. But, says Dr. Olshansky, we have already attained a true measure of immortality because our genetic material is passed on through sex from generation to generation. "Our immortality lies in our genes," he says.

All of this happens at a species level. Because humans are a sexually reproducing species, all humans, regardless of whether they reproduce, will die. A life of abstinence won't make you live longer. As the old joke goes, it will just feel like it.

This system benefits humankind in the long haul, albeit not necessarily you. Your one consolation is that the process of passing on your genes (that is, sex) is a whole lot of fun.

Talkin' about Evolution

The current life-death cycle leaves room for variety in the species, giving our genes the chance to adapt to an ever-changing environment, explains Dr. Olshansky. Each generation can adapt as the world changes and then can pass those adapted genes on to the next generation, he says.

There is a careful orchestration of all our living and dying. "The life spans of most species are linked to their reproductive periods," Dr. Olshansky says. "Mice and insects have short reproductive periods and very short lives. Humans, elephants, and turtles have long reproductive periods and, consequently, long life spans."

The connection is so strong that some researchers are even investigating how pushing back the reproductive period can extend life. "We've already done it with fruit flies," says Leonard Guarente, Ph.D., professor of biology at the Massachusetts Institute of Technology in Cambridge. "If you force them to mate late, over a few generations, you end up with flies that like mating late and that live longer."

But alas, they still age and die—and so do we—despite our best attempts to foil Mother Nature, says George Webster, Ph.D., researcher in molecular biology and aging in Satellite Beach, Florida, and author of *Hello, Methuselah!: Living to 100 and Beyond*. Biologists have determined that each cell in an organism will divide only so many times before it shuts down and becomes inactive, Dr. Webster says. What they haven't figured out yet is how cells decide when they're going to shut down.

The wear and tear of living also pushes this process along, says Siegfried Hekimi, Ph.D., professor of biology at McGill University in Montreal. "You accumulate defects from being alive," he says. "Cells get damaged. Cells wear out. You can slow this down, but there's no way to completely avoid it."

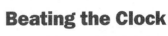

Beating the Clock

Okay, so death is inevitable. But dying before our

time is not. Granted, millions of men do make a hasty exit from the human race long before they're ready to pass the baton, but that's not because they're built that way. Often, they simply do things to accelerate the process.

The saying "live fast, die young" applies here, says Dr. Webster. "Men smoke. They eat fatty foods. They watch television. They sit around and don't exercise. They do all these wrong things. Then they end up with real trouble like heart disease or cancer and act like it's a sudden occurrence," he says. "Those diseases aren't a consequence of aging; they're a consequence of living poorly. Start laying plaque in your arteries, and you'll end up with heart disease. Injure your cells with toxins from cigarette smoke, and you'll get cancer."

And even if you somehow escape disease from the damage you've done, you may still accelerate the aging process, so you won't live as well or as long as you should have, adds Dr. Hekimi.

You can affect how long your cells continue to reproduce healthily by taking care of yourself, Dr. Hekimi says. "It's not like your clock is going tick, tock, tick, tock—bang!—you're dead." Your environment, especially your lifestyle, influences the ticking of that clock, he says.

"You know what to do to live as long as you're supposed to," Dr. Hekimi says. "Don't smoke. Drink in moderation. Be active, but don't overdo it. Don't work too hard. Don't eat garbage." Living to your maximum life span is mostly in your own hands. Experts can tell you what to do. But then you have to do the rest.

Out of Harm's Way

In a classic *Twilight Zone* episode, Roddy McDowall plays an astronaut who crash-lands on Mars, where he finds the inhabitants to be most accommodating. In fact, they're so darn nice that they build him an exact replica of his home back on Earth. McDowall is thrilled, until the walls slide up and he realizes to his horror that he's in a zoo.

This begs the question: What's so bad about that?

"The animals we take care of in captivity generally live longer in the habitats here than they do in the wild because we make sure that they have a good diet and are tended to when they're sick," says Victor Goldie, of the Docent Council at the Philadelphia Zoo. "And animals in the zoo are not subject to predation. Depending on the animal, the longer life span could be an additional couple of years to even decades."

If people lived in similar situations—where all their needs were seen to and they were kept from any dangerous environment—they, too, could live years longer, says James Enstrom, Ph.D., associate research professor in the School of Public Health at the University of California, Los Angeles.

The table below shows what happens when life's a real zoo.

Animal	Life Expectancy in the Wild	Potential Life Expectancy in Captivity
Lemur	12 to 20 years	Up to 30 years
Beaver	5 years	50 years
Elephant	35 years	70 years
Man (males)	74	85 years*

*Assumes that man lives a conservative lifestyle, which includes no tobacco, alcohol, caffeine, illegal drugs, or sexual promiscuity; dietary moderation; strong family and spiritual ties; and a commitment to education and being health-conscious. Yeah, it sounds like life in captivity to us.

How Long Do We Live?

What a Difference 100 Years Makes

When Jack London published *The Call of the Wild* in 1901, a man had to pack a whole lot of living into very few years. An average White male of the time could expect to live only to about 48. The average Black man died at just over 32. London himself made it only to 40—an age where many men today are just starting to get comfortable with life.

As the twentieth century gives its final curtain call, the average man doesn't have to worry about calling it curtains himself until he's into his eighth decade of life. During the past 100 years, we've essentially added almost another lifetime to the one we had.

Reeling In the Years

The most important contributors to the modern rise of life expectancy have been improved lifestyles and medical advances such as immunizations, which allow us to make it through the perilous period of growing up.

"Early in the century, infant and child mortality was remarkably high," says Dr. S. Jay Olshansky of the University of Chicago. "We've made remarkable progress in improving life expectancy this century by reducing infectious diseases among infants and children and reducing deaths among women during childbirth." By the time

Ed Sullivan was censoring Elvis Presley's gyrating hips in the 1950s, we had successfully developed vaccinations against some of our most crippling and deadly viral diseases, including polio, the measles, and rubella. We also greatly reduced the incidence of other killer diseases such as tuberculosis, smallpox, diphtheria, tetanus, and typhoid fever. As a result, life expectancy in midcentury rose to over 65 years for the average man.

Today, our problems catch up with us later in life, when our bodies slow down and stop working after years of wear and tear. The biggest foes that step between us and triple digits these days are heart disease, cancer, and stroke.

"These diseases are a multistep process," says David Smith, M.D., professor in the department of pathology and the Buehler Center on Aging at Northwestern University Medical School in Chicago. You didn't see much heart disease at the beginning of the century because people didn't live long enough to see the effects of damage done to their arteries, he says.

What has allowed men to add about seven years to their life expectancy in the latter half of this century has been a combination of medical advances and lifestyle changes such as healthier diets, reduced smoking and more exercise, Dr. Smith says. "There has been a 50 percent reduction in death as a result of heart disease from hardening of the arteries and stroke in the past 30 years. We're just starting to see the results of less smoking among men. And men are starting to improve their eating habits now as well," he says.

Home Free after 80

The United States may have a smaller proportion of men joining the club of octogenarians than Japan, where life expectancy is much longer than it is for most other folks on the globe. But studies show that if we can make it to the big eight-oh, we end up outliving 80-year-olds in Japan and many European countries.

If you want to increase your chances of making it into your seventies and beyond, the doctors from the esteemed Framingham Heart Study—a Massachusetts community-based health study of more than 10,000 men and women that has been in progress for more than 30 years—have a very simple prescription for men to follow: Smoke less, keep your blood pressure in check, and exercise to strengthen your lungs and lower your heart rate.

Among 747 healthy 50-year-old men whom researchers began studying more than two decades ago, those who had lower blood pressure, smoked fewer cigarettes, and had lower heart rates and better lung function—both associated with cardiovascular fitness—were significantly more likely to see their 75th birthday than those who did not.

The Outer Limits

So what's the longest you can expect to live once you've successfully navigated past childhood diseases, car crashes, and chronic diseases? Experts agree that you probably won't live as long as the oldest people on record—about 120.

The only authenticated case of a man who's ever reached this remarkable milestone was Shigechiyo Izumi, a Japanese man who made it to *The Guinness Book of World Records* for living 120 years and 237 days. More remarkably, Izumi continued to work until he was 105.

"Thousands of individuals will be able to make it past 100," says Dr. Olshansky. "But our

Men of Ages

Back in biblical times, longevity wasn't such a big deal. Heck, Moses lived 120 years without missing a step, according to the Bible. Noah kept trekking 350 years after the flood—living a colossal 950 years. And we hardly need mention Methuselah's claim to fame. At 969 years of age, he's credited with being the oldest man in history.

How'd they do it?

With all due respect, they most likely didn't. Theologians have mulled this question for years. By considering traditions of the time, they have developed very human explanations for what appear to be superhuman life spans.

"No one really has the answer, but there are two very plausible explanations," says the Reverend Glenn Asquith Jr., Ph.D., professor of pastoral theology at Moravian Theological Seminary in Bethlehem, Pennsylvania. "One is that the Israelites counted time differently. Some have theorized that they followed a lunar rather than a solar calendar."

An even better explanation is that the Israelites loved their heroes much in the way we do—by making them larger than life. It's like all of the embellishment surrounding George Washington, the Reverend Dr. Asquith says. "Most of these stories were passed down orally. So, with each telling, they likely became embellished. Since longevity was a sign of God's blessing to the ancient Israelites, it makes sense that they would make their heroes out to be ancient."

inherited program for growth and development leads inadvertently to a biological limit on life." Evidently, that's the price we pay for being a sexually reproducing species.

How Long Should We Live?

Testing the Limits

Reaching 100 years of age used to be so extraordinary that NBC weatherman Willard Scott devoted a few seconds of the *Today* show to wishing those long-lived "pretty ladies" and "fine gentlemen" much congratulations and continued health on that miraculous milestone. Nowadays, *Today* could devote half its air time to wishing 100-year-olds well.

Just in the 10 years between 1980 and 1990, the population of people older than 85 years increased by 40 percent. By 1990, there were about 30,000 people who lived past the 100-year mark. If we stay this course, researchers predict that by the time 2080 rolls around, there could be as many as 10 million centenarians. As this legion of graying Americans pushes into triple digits, it's likely that the record for maximum life span—currently set at 122 years—will be broken.

But where do we reach our limit?

It depends on whom you ask. There are two camps in the study of longevity. One believes that medical technology promises to churn out a future of modern-day Methuselahs. They contend that life expectancy, which is the estimated number of years that a person is expected to live on average, will reach 100 in the next generation. And soon, living to 200, 300, or more will not be out of the question. The second camp believes that all species have a genetic program for growth, development, and reproduction that inadvertently leads to a biological limit to life. As far as life expectancy goes, we've just about reached the practical limit, says Dr. S. Jay Olshansky of the University of Chicago.

Pushing the Envelope

Through a combination of curing chronic disease and controlling biological aging factors, the day will come when we live in an "ageless society," says Ronald Klatz, D.O., M.D., biomedical researcher and president of the American Academy of Anti-Aging Medicine in Chicago, one of the folks who believes that we've just begun to climb the ladder of longevity. "We won't suffer from degenerative diseases like heart disease and cancer that plague us today," he says. "We'll just die of total organ shutdown when our cells are no longer able to repair and reproduce. That's at least around age 160."

Just as splitting an atom was unthinkable in 1928 (but was accomplished in 1938), so will medical technology advance in ways we can't begin to imagine, adds Dr. George Webster, researcher in molecular biology and aging. "Each year, the National Library of Medicine receives about 1,700 reports on findings in biomedical research. Who ever imagined that we'd be able to clone a sheep? Yet it didn't take scientists long to figure that out," Dr. Webster says.

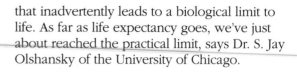

Scientists have already discovered genes that contribute to aging. They understand how hormones decline over time. They have a handle on how our DNA gets damaged through the years. They've studied ways to slow metabolism to prolong life. Now they just have to put it all together, says Dr. Webster. "We've been able to more than quadruple the life spans of worms by altering certain genes. Once we understand how these genes work, we can start producing substances that stop their action," he says. "If medical technology grows during the next 50 years at the pace it has grown during the past 50 years, we could push life expectancy into the hundreds. That's why I tell men of every age to start living healthfully, because if a 40-year-old or even 60-year-old man can make it another 25 years, he'll be able to reap the benefits of anti-aging medical technology."

Have We Hit the Ceiling?

And the Lord said, My spirit shall not always strive with man, for that he also is flesh: yet his days shall be an hundred and twenty years.
—**Genesis 6:3**

The Old Testament said it first. Skeptical scientists are still saying it today. It's not that they don't believe that hundreds of thousands of people will be celebrating their 100th birthdays in the years to come. But the buck pretty much stops there, they say.

"It's true that we're living about 30 years longer than we did at the beginning of the century," says Dr. Olshansky. "But if you look at the data, those advances are due to how much we've been able to lower infant and child mortality. Now that we're trying to extend life expectancy on the back end of life, those improvements have slowed dramatically."

In 1993, there was actually a small dip in life expectancy, followed by a stagnant period in 1994. Since then, we've made some gains. Life expectancy is expected to pick up some steam again, but the U.S. Census Bureau has conservative estimates. By 2050, they predict, the average man will add about 7 years to his life, living to about 79.7 years. If they're

Life Span versus Life Expectancy

Contrary to what you might think, life expectancy charts don't tell you much about how long you, specifically, have to live. They predict how long you, your next-door neighbor, the president, Larry Bird, and a million other men have to live—72.4 years—but that's only on average.

Your life *span*, meanwhile, is how long you actually live—and that could be anywhere from 60 to 120 years. And if you're in much better physical shape than the average Joe your age, chances are that your life span will be higher than the life expectancy. "The life span of an individual may turn out to be very different from the life expectancy. You may die tomorrow, or you could live to be more than 100 years old," says Dr. David Smith of Northwestern University Medical School. "At times when life spans are changing rapidly, life expectancies have little predictive value for the life span of an individual. Life expectancies are a prediction of what is to occur in the distant future yet are based on data from people who have recently died, so they are not very relevant to people living or being born today," explains Dr. Smith. In other words, just because the chart says 72 doesn't mean that you should schedule yourself to die then.

right, plenty of men would reach the century mark, but not much longer than that.

"Though people like to talk about how much we understand the aging process, that doesn't mean that we'll be able to do anything about it," says Dr. Siegfried Hekimi of McGill University. "We can mutate certain genes in worms so that they live five times longer, but that's by slowing them down metabolically so that they live five times slower. You have to stop living to stop aging, and I doubt that people want to do that."

Untimely Endings

Why We Don't Live As Long As We Should

Comic actor John Candy. Professional baseball player Nolan Ryan. At age 43, both hit milestones in their lives. One had just pitched two no-hitters, putting the finishing touches on a glorious major-league career that spanned 27 years. The other smoked and had a weight problem and was dead of a heart attack. Sometimes our destiny isn't in our hands. But sometimes it is.

Lots of guys point their fingers at the fates when talking about their health, says Walter M. Bortz II, M.D., clinical associate professor of medicine at Stanford University School of Medicine and author of *Dare to Be 100.* Or worse, they believe that coming from "good stock" gives them license for self-abuse. The truth is that our genes generally have less to do with how long we live than we'd like to believe, says Dr. Bortz. "Genetics have about a 20 percent influence on life span," he says. "The rest is in your hands."

"The length of your life is hugely affected by your lifestyle," agrees Dr. George Webster, researcher in molecular biology and aging. "Lots of people today are living a hell of a long time because they're finally doing what they ought to be doing—not smoking, getting out of their chairs, and becoming more active." Here are the top seven behaviors experts say will shorten your life and what you can do about them.

The Meat-and-Potato Men

Sixty-nine percent of men admit that they struggle with eating a balanced diet. Most of us eat about 10 percent more than the 30-percent-calories-from-fat-a-day plan we're supposed to stick to. We're eating a measly three or four servings of fruits and vegetables each day instead of the five to nine the U.S. Department of Agriculture Food Guide Pyramid recommends. And about one-third of men are overweight. "Then we're surprised when our health gives out," Dr. Webster says.

"We need to and can do much better," says Ken Goldberg, M.D., founder and director of the Male Health Institute in Dallas and author of *How Men Can Live As Long As Women.* "The key is to follow a healthy diet most of the time, so you can have nachos and beer at the ball game and it won't matter." Here's what experts recommend.

Eat just one. If each time you eat, you include a fruit or a vegetable, you'll steadily improve your health, says Dr. Goldberg. The 30-year Framingham Heart Study by Harvard researchers found that with each additional serving of fruits and vegetables that 832 men ages 45 to 65 ate, the lower their risk of stroke became. And that's only one benefit. Eating more fruits and vegetables also lowers your risk for colon cancer and heart disease, adds Dr. Goldberg.

Get the red out. When faced with a choice in meats, choose fish, turkey, or chicken, Dr. Goldberg says. A landmark study of close to 48,000 male health professionals found that men who ate the most red meat had a significantly higher risk for advanced prostate cancer than those who ate the least.

Stop, drop, and live. A side benefit of eating more fruits and vegetables and less fatty red meat is that you'll also likely shed a few pounds, says Dr. Goldberg. Even the least bit of waist-whittling can add to your life. In another landmark, 22-year study of nearly 20,000 men, researchers found that being just 2 to 6 percent over your ideal weight increases your risk for cardiovascular disease. Being as much as 20 percent over increases your risk by more than 2½ times that of ideal-weight men.

The Benchwarmers

In the game of life, more than half of all men are benchwarmers, says the American Heart Association (AHA). That means that more than 50 percent of men don't get moving for a minimum of a half-hour a day, three days a week.

That's a sin, Dr. Goldberg says. "Studies show that exercise may be more effective at heading off an early death than quitting smoking, losing weight, or stopping drinking," he says. Here are some tips for getting in gear.

Prevent the big "C." After studying 47,723 male doctors for six years, Harvard researchers found that men who got the most exercise had only half the risk for colon cancer as those who got the least. So do your colon a favor by exercising for 30 minutes at least three times a week, recommends Dr. Goldberg.

Aim for gains. It doesn't matter what your fitness level is when you start. It matters that you improve, says Dr. Goldberg. Researchers at the Cooper Institute for Aerobics Research studied the effects of increasing fitness levels on 10,000 men over a five-year period. Men who improved their fitness level enough to run a minute longer than their original treadmill time also had a lower death rate than those who stayed unfit. In fact, every one-minute increase in maximum treadmill time equaled an impressive 8 percent drop in risk of death.

"You should constantly challenge yourself to improve your fitness level," says Dr. Goldberg. If your exercise of choice is walking or running, try to increase your speed or your distance every few months, he suggests.

Decline the decline. As you age, it's likely that your physical performance will decrease over time, and the more that performance decreases, the more susceptible you can be to disease. You can slow that decline simply by exercising more, says Dr. Bortz. After about age 30, people who exercise start to see only a 0.5 percent decline in performance each year, he says. "Unfit folks of the same age see a 2 percent decline. That means the man who exercises will have surrendered only about 15 percent of his vital capacity by the time he's 65; the nonexerciser, 70 percent."

Hard-Hearted Men

The AHA estimates that more than 30 percent of men ages 45 to 54, more than 40 percent of men ages 55 to 64, and more than 55 percent of men ages 65 to 74 have high blood pressure. Making matters worse, about 50 percent of men in this country have cholesterol levels higher than 200 milligrams per deciliter. And that's just the numbers that have been reported. Many men are never diagnosed.

"There's just no excuse," says Ichiro Kawachi, M.D., Ph.D., associate professor of health and social behavior at the Harvard School of Public Health. "These are conditions that are easily detected and treated." Here are some things you can do yourself to minimize the damage.

Burn your arteries clean. Playing half-court hoops for 30 minutes a day can raise your levels of "good" high-density lipoprotein (HDL) cholesterol by as much as 6 milligrams per deciliter. A group of Spanish researchers has found that, on average, for every 100 calories you burn a day, your levels of artery-clearing HDL cholesterol rise by about 2 milligrams per deciliter.

Go low. Researchers from several U.S. cities put 459 folks on a low-fat diet chock-full of fruits, vegetables, grains, and low-fat dairy products. After eight weeks, those with high blood pressure saw their systolic pressure (the top number) drop an average of 11.4 points and their diastolic pressure (the bottom number) dip an average of 5.5 points. This may sound like a lot to swallow, but the famous Food Guide Pyramid recommends eating 2 to 3 servings of dairy products, 3 to 5 servings of vegetables, 2 to 4 servings of fruits, and 6 to 11 servings of grains every day.

The Smoking Man

"Smoking is the single most identifiable and strongest factor for a shortened life span," says Dr. James Enstrom of the University of California, Los Angeles, who has spent more than a decade studying the effects of lifestyle on the health of Mormons. Yet 26 million American men are still puffing away, according to the AHA. If you want to beat death by smoke inhalation, here's what you need to do.

Don't start. A British study says it best: When comparing the longevity prospects of 1,624 men who never smoked against 3,151 lifetime smokers, researchers found that, based on death rates, only an estimated 42 percent of the smokers would live to be 73, compared to 78 percent of the nonsmokers.

Kick the habit. The best thing a smoker can do for himself is to put out his cigarette—for good, says Dr. Kawachi. After quitting for just two weeks to three months, your lung function increases up to 30 percent. And after 10 smoke-free years, your risk of dying from lung cancer

The Seven Not-So-Deadly Sins

Thanks to Sunday school, we know all about the Seven Deadly Sins. But just how deadly are those sins? The *British Medical Journal* (*BMJ*) posed that question to experts in the health field. If properly directed, it turns out that some of those "sins" can actually help us live longer. Used wrongly, though, they can kill us—kind of like booze. Here's what the experts said. Pick your poison.

Lust: There are 3 million to 5 million new cases of chlamydia annually. Add to that the millions of new cases of other sexually transmitted diseases, and you have a healthy case against lust. But when push comes to shove, lust drives us to plant our seeds and keep the gene line immortal, writes Liam Farrell, M.D., a general practitioner at Crossmaglen Health Centre in Crossmaglen, Ireland, in the *BMJ*.

Envy: Envy has been posited as the core emotion that drives us to murder. If that's the case, we have it to blame for about 20,000 deaths a year. Sometimes called "an unpleasant thought wrapped in an unwanted emotion," envy has nothing good going for it. Let's pick another vice.

Wrath: Angry, wrathful emotions can increase heart disease risk by two- or threefold. Properly directed, though, wrath can empower the masses to right wrongs such as slavery and oppression, writes Simon Chapman, M.D., associate professor of public health and community medicine at the University of Sydney.

Pride: Pride seems to rank at the bottom of the list of "sins to be really concerned about." But lack of pride—

is similar to that of a nonsmoker. Here's a tip to help you quit: If you decide to go cold turkey, be sure to resist cheating on the first day. One study by the Duke University Nico-

by way of low self-esteem—is blamed for many of society's ills these days. Take drug abuse, alcoholism, suicide, eating disorders, depression, and racism, for example. All of these often have low self-esteem at their core. Well-earned pride has been associated with "happiness, satisfaction, loving, and being loved," notes Simon Wessely, M.D., of the department of psychological medicine at King's College School of Medicine and Dentistry in London.

Gluttony: Not to point any fingers, but about one-third of men are overweight. Being seriously overweight puts you at risk for heart disease, stroke, and diabetes, just to name a few. This makes gluttony—if that's your vice—a seriously deadly sin.

Sloth: This sin, argues James McCormick, M.D., professor in the department of community health and general practice at Trinity College in Dublin, is one we might consider taking up, if it means slowing down. But he also notes that sloth has literally become a deadly sin for those "couch potatoes" whose idea of exercise is occasionally shuffling the sofa cushions to search for the remote control.

Greed: Let's face it, a little greed has been a big motivator for inventors, scientists, and artists. As for how deadly it is, it's hard to say. But greed can make you lonely and miserly, even as it drives some people to hurt those who get in their way. Take Ebenezer Scrooge, whose avarice would have meant the end of Tiny Tim, had Scrooge not seen the light. And remember, Scrooge's life was a lonely, friendless one, while his greed consumed him.

tine Research program in Durham, North Carolina, found that those who already sneaked a butt on day one were 10 times more likely to be smoking six months later.

Cut back now. Though quitting is the way to go, even cutting down can do some good, says Dr. Kawachi. Researchers of the Framingham Heart Study report that one of the benchmarks of making it to age 75 is fewer cigarettes smoked per day among those who smoke. It's not a perfect solution, but it's better than nothing. "Very few smokers, in fact, succeed in cutting down," says Dr. Kawachi. "The nature of nicotine addiction is such that most smokers end up going back up to their previous levels." (In pharmacology, this phenomenon is known as tolerance.) So it's better to quit altogether than to attempt a halfway solution, says Dr. Kawachi. "Also, don't believe tobacco industry advertisements about 'low-nicotine' or 'low-tar' cigarettes. There is no evidence that smoking these brands results in lower levels of harmful substances in the body, or lower risks of death and disease," he adds.

Type A-ngry

Cardiologists used to say that being a high-pressured, ladder-climbing, positively type A kind of guy was enough to put you in your own risk category for an early departure. In one study of 1,305 men, Harvard researchers found that anger caused a two- to threefold increase in risk for heart disease. Here's how to take the edge off.

Move into management. Though more research needs to be done, Dr. Kawachi believes that men who are frequently angry could lower their heart attack risk by learning how to better control their anger, for example, through an anger-management workshop.

Take a breath. If you're the kind of guy who can't wait for others to finish their sentences before you chime in, you might find yourself part of fewer conversations in the long run. After tracking 750 men, researchers found that the domineering types were 60 percent more likely to die during the study than their quieter counterparts. Learning relaxation techniques may not only make you a better conversationalist but also help you live longer, says Dr. Kawachi.

The Disengagers

It's natural that we die at 75, says Dr. Bortz, especially since so many men are preparing themselves for death the minute they retire. "With the turn of a page on a calendar, we feel rendered obsolete. There's nothing wrong with retiring at 65, or at 45 for that matter, but it is imperative to feel necessary," Dr. Bortz says. The key is to make sure that you stay engaged in life in your later adult years the same way you were in your early adult years. Here's how.

Stand at attention. "It's a fact that many men develop problems with erections in their later years," Dr. Goldberg says. In fact, some 10 million to 15 million men have trouble with impotence.

If you're suffering an erection problem, it may not be permanent, says Dr. Goldberg. Many cases of impotence are the result of side effects from medication or sometimes simply from psyching yourself out, he says. The point is that you won't know unless you get it checked out.

Graduate. After each big stage in your life, there is something that follows, says Dr. Bortz. You graduate from high school; you go to college. You graduate from college; you get a job. Well, plan something after you "graduate" from your job, he says. Take your skills on the road and volunteer. Or map out the places you want to visit. "Too often, the paycheck goes, the

self-esteem goes, the erection goes, and the man goes. Don't fall into that trap. You would never stop dreaming and making plans at 35. Don't do it at 65, or you might be stuck dying for 30 years."

The Exam-Skippers

As often as you skipped your 8:00 A.M. sociology class in school, you likely still had the sense to show up on exam day so that you wouldn't flunk out. Though you're not getting graded on life, the test of the quality of life is often your health. Routine medical exams can make sure that you ace it.

Yet men continue to skip their exams. In one study of 897 men older than 65, only 67 percent reported ever having a digital rectal examination, the first line of defense in detecting and preventing advanced prostate cancer. When asked why they hadn't submitted to the test, many said that it was because they hadn't had a problem. "Men must remember that the time to catch problems is before you know you have them," says Dr. Goldberg. "That's when they're treatable." Here are a couple of ways to prepare for your next exam.

Do it yourself. Everyone should give his body a once-over every month for changes like lumps in the chest, testicles, armpits, or neck; persistent unhealed sores on the skin or in the mouth; and skin discoloration or changes in moles as well as keeping an eye out for changes in heart rate, urine or bowel movements, and energy levels, Dr. Goldberg says.

Take the tests. You know those maintenance schedules listed in the back of your car manual? You can (and should) treat yourself to your own. (See Medical Testing on page 62 for a full list of tests you need throughout your life.) Generally, doctors recommend about 19 routine medical tests to screen a man's health. Most need to be done every three years before age 40 and about every two years after that.

Life: Quality versus Quantity

Living It to the Max

There are times, to be sure, when it seems that Mark Twain hit the nail right on the head when he wrote: "The only way to keep your health is to eat what you don't want, drink what you don't like, and do what you'd druther not."

But it's precisely that kind of Pudd'n-headed thinking that has been driving men to an early grave for too long. So, just for the record, you don't have to give up everything that makes life worth living in order to live a long life.

"Guys like to say, 'I don't want to live forever anyway,' as they smoke their cigarettes and eat their fatty foods," says Royda Crose, Ph.D., associate professor and associate director of the Fisher Institute for Wellness at Ball State University in Muncie, Indiana, and author of *Why Women Live Longer Than Men.* "But when they reach an age they used to consider old, they're not any more ready to die than they were before. And they sure don't say, 'Gee, I'm glad I smoked all those cigarettes and ate all those burgers because now I have emphysema and arteriosclerosis,'" says Dr. Crose.

When it comes to life, the choice is not quantity versus quality, says Dr. Ken Goldberg of the Male Health Institute. You can have it both ways. The idea is not to extend life for the sake of living longer but to be able to have sex, play golf, travel, and enjoy life right up to the very end, he says. "If you're willing to make some changes, that can be for a very long time," Dr. Goldberg says.

You don't have to make New Year's resolutions like "I'll never eat a cheese steak again." "Small changes, like taking the stairs instead of the elevator and getting enough sleep, can make big differences for the average person," says Dr. James Enstrom of the University of California, Los Angeles. Aside from the lifestyle changes you hear about all the time, there are loads of honestly enjoyable ways you can make your life happier, healthier, and longer. Here are a few to try.

Living the Sporting Life

Take up a sport, suggests Dr. Goldberg. Almost any sport will do, he says. Recruit some friends to play with on a regular basis. And chances are good that you'll still be living the sporting life all the way into your seventies, if not beyond.

A team of Swedish researchers studied the effects of regular activity throughout life on the physical ability of 233 men at age 76. The volunteers were asked to describe their involvement in competitive sports, recreational sports, occupational physical work, and household work as well as their means of transportation during five periods of their lives, beginning at age 10. The men who had the highest levels of activity after age 35 were the most mobile at 76. And the best activity for ensuring that you'll still be brisk at three-quarters of a century is playing recreational sports.

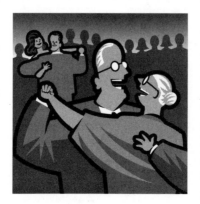

Regular physical activity has been linked to lower rates of high blood pressure, diabetes, osteoporosis, colon cancer, anxiety, and depression. Men who get their duffs in motion for close to a half-hour most days of the week actually have about half the risk for heart disease that sedentary men can expect.

It's never too late to start.

(continued on page 16)

How Long Do You Have?

This chart, developed by Michael F. Roizen, M.D., chair of the department of anesthesia and critical care at the University of Chicago, and author of *RealAge: Are You As Young As You Can Be?*, will give you a rough idea of how many years you have left. To estimate how long you'll live, begin by using the table at right to find the median life expectancy of your age group. Then add or subtract years based on the risk factors listed below.

	Gain in Life Expectancy		
HEALTH	**+3 YEARS**	**+2 YEARS**	**+1 YEAR**
Blood pressure	Between 90/65 and 120/81	Less than 90/65 without heart disease	Between 121/82 and 129/85
Diabetes	N/A	N/A	N/A
Total cholesterol	N/A	N/A	Less than 160
HDL cholesterol	N/A	N/A	More than 55
Compared with that of others my age, my health is:	N/A	N/A	Excellent
LIFESTYLE	**+3 YEARS**	**+2 YEARS**	**+1 YEAR**
Cigarette smoking	None	Ex-smoker, no cigarettes for more than 5 years	Ex-smoker, no cigarettes for 3–5 years
Exercise average	More than 90 minutes per day of exercise for more than 3 years	More than 60 minutes per day for more than 3 years	More than 20 minutes per day for more than 3 years
Saturated fat in diet	N/A	Less than 7%	7%–10%
Fruits and vegetables	N/A	N/A	5 servings per day
FAMILY	**+3 YEARS**	**+2 YEARS**	**+1 YEAR**
Marital status	N/A	Happily married man	N/A
Disruptive events in the past year†	N/A	N/A	N/A
Social groups, friends seen more than once a month‡	N/A	Three	Two
Parents' age of death	N/A	N/A	Both lived past 75

*A pack-year is one pack per day for a year.
†Deaths of family members, job changes, moves, lawsuits, financial insecurity, etc.
‡People who offer support through disruptive events (applicable only in case of two or more such events).
SOURCE: Michael F. Roizen, M.D., using data abstracted from the Real Age and Age-Reduction-Planning programs of Medical Informatics.

Age	Male	Scoring Risk Factors
20–59	73	Use table as shown
60–69	76	Reduce loss or gain by 20%
70–79	78	Reduce loss or gain by 50%
80+	Add 5 years to current age	Reduce loss or gain by 75%

Start with Your Median Life Expectancy

No Change ┌──────── **Loss in Life Expectancy** ────────┐

No Change	–1 YEAR	–2 YEARS	–3 YEARS	TALLY
130/86	Between 131/87 and 140/90	Between 141/91 and 150/95	More than 151/96	_____
None	Type II (adult-onset)	N/A	Type I (juvenile-onset)	_____
161–200	201–240	241–280	More than 280	_____
45–54	40–44	Less than 40	N/A	_____
Very good or fair	N/A	Bad	Poor	_____

No Change	–1 YEAR	–2 YEARS	–3 YEARS	TALLY
Ex-smoker, no cigarettes for 1–3 years	Ex-smoker, no cigarettes for 5 months–1 year	Smoker, 0–20 pack-years*	Smoker, more than 20 pack-years	_____
More than 10 minutes per day for more than 3 years	More than 5 minutes per day for more than 3 years	Less than 5 minutes per day	None	_____
10%–13%	N/A	More than 13%	N/A	_____
N/A	None	N/A	N/A	_____

No Change	–1 YEAR	–2 YEARS	–3 YEARS	TALLY
Widowed man	Divorced man	Divorced woman	Single man	_____
N/A	One	Two	Three	_____
One	N/A	None	N/A	_____
One lived past 75	N/A	N/A	Neither lived past 75	_____

Your estimated life expectancy _____

A study of almost 10,000 men found that those who became fit during a five-year period had about half the risk of dying from any cause compared to those who stayed out of shape. "Even making small changes like walking briskly to the bus stop, mowing the lawn without a riding mower, and climbing the stairs at work can make a difference," says Dr. Goldberg. On the other hand, by choosing absolute inactivity, you can shave almost six years off your life span, according to findings from a study of 27,000 people by researchers in California.

Finally, studies show what we've known since the days of the recess bell: Taking time to go out and play can sure take the edge off a stressful day.

Curiouser and Curiouser

Researchers from Menlo Park, California, who conducted a five-year study of 1,118 men between ages 60 and 86 found that those who were still alive at the end of the study had significantly higher levels of curiosity than those who had died during the same time.

Curiosity is not only a driving force that keeps your gray matter stoked, but maintained over time, it can also help you find suitable ways to cope through the myriad challenges that life throws your way as you age, says Gary E. Swan, Ph.D., director of the Center for Health Sciences at SRI International (formerly Stanford Research Institute) in Menlo Park. "Older adults should attend as many continuing education classes as possible because they provide the environmental support for you to solve problems creatively, to try new things, and to listen to new ideas," Dr. Swan advises.

Don't Take My Wife, Please

Comedians have been getting cheap laughs at the expense of the old ball and chain for as long as there have been women and steel. The funny thing is that as much as we joke about women driving us to our graves, the fact is that they actually add years to our lives. Finding a mate and being happily married is about as good as, if not better for our health than, quitting smoking, maintaining healthy blood pressure, eating a low-fat diet, or exercising more than 60 minutes a day.

Marriage may also be the key to disease survival, say experts. When researchers at the Veterans Administration Medical Center in Miami checked the survival rates of 143,969 men with prostate cancer, they found that those who were married lived almost three years longer than those who either were never married or were separated or divorced. Marriage is even better for your health if you do it only once. Researchers found that the trauma of divorce can be bad enough to negate the benefits of being remarried.

"But the findings are pretty consistent that being married has plenty of health benefits for men," says study author Joan Tucker, Ph.D., assistant professor of psychology at Brandeis University in Waltham, Massachusetts. "Women traditionally do things for men that have health benefits. Things like improving his diet, reducing his risky behavior, providing stress relief, and helping him remember to take medication are all strong health supports."

You Are What You Eat

Remember the tired old "an apple a day" cliché? Well, a 20-some-year study of almost 10,000 people in Finland confirmed it. Those who ate the most flavonoids, which are natural antioxidants found in many fruits and vegetables, had lower risks for all cancers and half the risk for lung cancer than those who ate the least. The clear winner for lowering lung cancer rates? You guessed it: apples.

But apples aren't the only fruit of paradise for your health. A study of more than

2,000 Welsh men demonstrated that those who ate the most of any kind of fruit had half the risk for all cancers compared to those who ate the least.

Hell, it's becoming so hip to eat healthy that major-league ballpark stadiums are even hawking fruits and vegetables next to the weenies and fries these days. Busch Stadium, the Astrodome, Dodger Stadium, Jacobs Field, Oriole Park at Camden Yards, Riverfront Stadium, and Shea Stadium all offer vegetables, garden salads, or fruit and vegetable platters. Others, including Candlestick Park and Wrigley Field, offer garden burgers and other healthful stadium snacks.

Laughing in the Face of Death

Though Bobby McFerrin almost drove us all to an early grave in 1988, with his incessant and insipid "Don't Worry, Be Happy," his advice was scientifically sound. If you can laugh in the face of adversity, you can live better, longer.

A Japanese researcher studying 157 men and women ages 65 and older has found a strong connection between maintaining a general sense of well-being and having low levels of total cholesterol, low levels of artery-blocking low-density lipoprotein (LDL) cholesterol, and high levels of healthful high-density lipoprotein (HDL) cholesterol. Lifting your spirits, he concluded, is important in caring for your heart.

Any moves that men can make to relieve their stress and lighten their moods will probably decrease their risks for heart attack, says Dr. Ichiro Kawachi of the Harvard School of Public Health.

You, Too, Can Live Fast and Die Young

When it comes to lifestyle, lots of guys think they're Mr. Rock-and-Roll.

Statistically speaking, you don't see people who make a habit of abusing themselves make it through unscathed, says John J. Mulvihill, M.D., professor of human genetics and founder of the cancer genetics program at the University of Pittsburgh. More likely, you'll go the way of other men who picked the fast lane and passed their contemporaries on their way to the grave. The following are some examples you might not want to follow.

Jimi Hendrix—Mr. 'Scuse-Me-While-I-Kiss-the-Sky was once quoted as saying, "Knowing me, I'll probably get busted at my own funeral." Close. It caught up with him at age 27 when, after partying all night, he took too many sleeping pills. It wasn't the pills that did him in, though. He got sick in the night and suffocated on his own vomit.

Jerry Garcia—This Grateful Dead guru is the classic tale of too little, too late. A long-time abuser of heroin, LSD, and other drugs, Garcia, who was also quite overweight, had an enlarged heart, and had diabetes by the time he was 44. Though he cut back on cigarettes and drugs and tried to get in shape after that, he still struggled with addiction and his health. He died of a heart attack at a drug treatment center at age 53.

James Dean—Dean left this world violently in a high-speed crash while cruising a California highway in "The Little Bastard," a gray Porsche he liked enough to name. Ironically, earlier that year Dean had filmed a commercial for safe driving, saying, "Take it easy drivin', uh, the life you save might be mine, you know?"

The Gender Gap

Why Do Women Live Longer?

In 1940, the average woman lived 65.2 years; the average man, 60.8—a difference of a little more than 4 years. Over the course of the century that gap has widened to about 7 years. And though it appears that males are making slight headway—the National Center for Health Statistics currently predicts that women will outlive men by only 6.4 years—the fact remains that men still die more often and earlier than women from all leading causes of death, especially heart disease, cancer, and accidents.

When asked why he's likely to die sooner, a man may blame his lot in life. He works harder; he has more stress. It only makes sense that he'll die sooner. Doctors specializing in men's health, however, say that's not quite the case. "It's because men are not involved with their health and their bodies the way women are," explains Dr. Ken Goldberg of the Male Health Institute. "And it's killing us."

Sex Ed

To be fair, women receive training about their bodies at a very early age, says Dr. Royda Crose of Ball State University. Women menstruate. They need an annual checkup when using birth control such as the Pill or a diaphragm. Going to the doctor and being in touch with their bodies is a much larger fact of their lives.

There are no such parallels for men. There's no checkup required at the convenience store to buy condoms. And though men go through

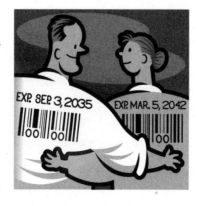

changes during puberty, too, not many get a heart-to-heart from their fathers about wet dreams, Dr. Crose says.

Even worse, men often get the message that they should be invincible loners and that it's not manly to take care of yourself, Dr. Goldberg says.

Ironically, men who beat the averages handle old age a whole lot better than their female counterparts, says Dr. Ichiro Kawachi of the Harvard School of Public Health. "Older women often spend the last years of their lives with more debilitation than men of the same age," Dr. Kawachi says.

The key to living longer is to live a little more like a woman, Dr. Goldberg says—which, we rush to point out, doesn't mean sacrificing any of your manhood. "I'm talking about men like Michael Jordan, who take care of themselves and live quality, healthy lives," he says. "Men need to hear more about what they should do for themselves to not just live longer but be able to keep their health right up until the time they die. That's what's important."

Turn Your Head and Cough

Maybe it's because our first introduction to physical examinations was being groped and told to cough by a school nurse known as the Claw, but men have a problem going to the doctor. Women make about 130 million more visits to the doctor each year than men.

"Men believe that they're bulletproof, and like most people, they're afraid that the doctor will find something wrong with them," Dr. Goldberg says. And that's the kicker because having your doctor find something wrong with you often is a very good thing. "If a doctor catches the problem before you feel bad from it, that means that it's usually early enough to cure it," he says.

Preventive maintenance. It's a term we all know but one we usually associate with our cars, not our bodies. Most guys wouldn't wait until they heard that horrible grinding sound before getting their car's brakes checked, Dr. Goldberg says. By then it's a whole lot more expensive to fix than just replacing the pads. "Your body is the same way. Better to bring down high cholesterol than perform a double bypass," Dr. Goldberg says.

If you want to help close the seven-year longevity lead that women have on us, you're going to have to start practicing prevention and getting more in touch with your body. Here's your action plan.

Search your tree. Lots of the top men-killing diseases run in families. Prostate cancer, colon cancer, heart disease, and testicular cancer are all deep-rooted conditions that, if caught early, are easily nipped in the bud, says Dr. Goldberg. "If you know your family history and get the appropriate tests, you can avoid or treat these conditions entirely," he says.

Put yourself to the test. Thanks to the media, every man knows that women should do monthly breast self-examinations. But how many men know to check their own testicles? "Testicular cancer is the number one solid cancer in males younger than 35," Dr. Goldberg says. "Every man who has reached puberty should examine his testicles once a month." It's best to check them in the shower, where the warm water relaxes the scrotum. Run your fingers around the circumference; you're looking for lumps or hard spots. The testicle should feel like a hard-boiled egg without the shell, says Dr. Goldberg.

Transsexual Salvation?

If women live about seven years longer than men, does that mean that your average Joe could up his life span by becoming your (not-so-)average Josephine? In short, would you live longer if you underwent a sex change?

"Theoretically, you might see an improvement in cholesterol levels because of the effects of estrogen," says Walter J. Meyer III, M.D., vice dean of the School of Medicine at the University of Texas Medical Branch at Galveston, where they have one of the nation's longest continuously running gender clinics. Also, a decrease in male hormones linked to negative emotions such as anger could result in a lower risk for heart disease. Research shows that when men are deprived of androgens (male hormones) they feel significantly less anger and aggression.

But frankly, there just aren't enough people who have changed genders to know, says Dr. Meyer.

Besides, the stress and trauma surrounding changing your sex would likely offset any physical benefits, says Dr. Royda Crose of Ball State University. "If you're happy as a man, it's best to change your behaviors rather than your anatomy."

Dr. Goldberg recommends making a health appointment with yourself the first of every month (or a day that's easy to remember, like when you pay the mortgage) to give yourself the following once-over.

- Check your skin for unusual growths, changes, or sores.
- Check your chest around the nipples for lumps; men can get breast cancer, too.
- Check the glands in your neck, armpits, and groin for swelling.

- Check your resting heart rate. Significant changes can signal the beginning of heart disease.

Check in with the doc. Find a physician whom you honestly like—a guy you trust and can talk to. And see him once a year. It's the single best thing you can do for yourself, Dr. Goldberg says. "It's not just a matter of keeping you alive longer. It's keeping you healthy longer so that you can play sports, have sex, and enjoy life no matter what age you are."

Living Dangerously

Close to 95,000 men a year die of lung cancer, compared to 66,000 women. Nearly twice as many men as women die of cirrhosis of the liver. And males are three times as likely to be killed in accidents. The reasons are obvious. Men smoke more, drink more, and take more unnecessary risks than women.

"Add to that the fact that men eat more meat, fat, dairy products, eggs, and high-calorie foods than women, while women eat more fruits, vegetables, whole grains, and low-calorie foods," says Dr. Crose. "It's small wonder that men's lives are cut short."

And cut is exactly the word to describe the often sudden ends that men come to, says Dr. Kawachi. "The biggest killer of men in their prime is heart attack. Men also die of sudden death more frequently than women. They have no inkling that they have heart disease, then they get ventricular fibrillation and drop dead," he says.

One way to avoid getting stopped in your tracks is to have annual physicals. Another is to make small lifestyle adjustments to keep healthier and safer. Here are doctors' top tips.

Terminate tobacco. Whether you chew it or smoke it, tobacco use dramatically raises your risk for cancer, Dr. Goldberg says. Chewing tobacco causes oral cancer. Smoking is responsible for almost 90 percent of lung cancers among men and significantly raises a person's risk for developing cancer of the pancreas, kidney, bladder, and esophagus.

"People tire of hearing it, but quitting smoking is the best thing you can do for yourself," Dr. Kawachi says. "If you're a lifetime smoker, you have a one in four chance of dying from a disease related to that habit, especially before age 65." No matter how old you are when you quit, you lower your risk of cancer and heart disease almost immediately, Dr. Kawachi says. Research shows that your risk of having a heart attack drops within the first 24 hours. And within the first five years, your risk of dying from lung cancer is cut in half.

Drink, but think. Once you have a few, you're well past the point of thinking about your drinking. So try doing what women—who are frequently designated drivers—do. Before you start, think about what you're going to drink and what you're going to do afterward. Then limit yourself to just a couple. "While there's evidence that moderate drinking may be good for the heart, excessive booze is bad for it. Plus it increases your risk for cancer and cirrhosis of the liver," Dr. Goldberg says. Booze is partly to blame for five times as many men as women drowning, though more men know how to swim, and for men being almost 2½ times more likely to die in a car accident than women, he says.

Flip-flop fiber and fat. Most men eat more fat than they should, and they're often eating more than they realize. To get less artery-clogging fat in your diet, make a point to choose fibrous foods over fatty foods whenever possible, says Dr. Kawachi. That means if there's a choice between a baked potato and fries, go with the baked potato.

"This is often harder for men than for women," Dr. Crose says. "Women become concerned about food at an early age, which is a problem regarding eating disorders, but it can be helpful in preventing chronic diseases later in life." By keeping this rule in mind, you'll almost automatically eat more fruits, vegetables, and grains and less processed, high-fat foods.

Angry Young Men

There's increasing evidence that angry young men don't grow up to be angry old men. They die before they get the chance.

"High levels of anger are a big risk for heart attack," Dr. Kawachi says. "The relative risk of having negative emotions like anger and anxiety are almost as strong as other risk factors like high cholesterol. And men are particularly at risk."

This also is one area in which testosterone—the hormone that gives you many of the male characteristics you enjoy (such as your sex drive)—is not your best ally, experts say. Testosterone increases aggression. You need to be aware of it and manage it, Dr. Crose says. Here's how.

Play ball! Here's a health tip that you can take to heart. Go shoot some hoops, join a softball league, or play any sport you like with a bunch of other men. "Sports can be very beneficial for men because it's one arena that gives men freedom to show emotions that they may not be able to show in other parts of their lives," Dr. Crose says. "Men can release there. They can hug each other. And if things get intense enough, they're even allowed to cry."

Make a connection. Friends are good for your health. "Unfortunately, men tend to rely on women for their socialization," Dr. Crose says. "That doesn't give them anyone to talk to of the same sex who may be going through the same things. It generally takes a crisis before men will reach out and talk to other men. Make friends, lighten up, and talk to one another—right now. You only have one life. It's better with some friends."

Sex and Death

Fancy cars, flowers, and expensive dinners are pretty normal parts of human courting behavior that are well-known for cutting a hunk out of a man's paycheck, if not occasionally his ego. But does all of this courting also take a slice off his life? One British geneticist thinks so.

"It's well-established in many species that in absence of mating behavior, males live much longer," says David Gems, Ph.D., researcher in the department of biology at University College London. "Castration increases longevity in a variety of vertebrates. Neutering tomcats has an enormous impact on their life expectancy."

Dr. Gems himself found that male worms lived up to twice as long when kept by themselves, as opposed to living with other males or with females. That's because they spent so much energy mating or attempting to mate that it shortened their lives, Dr. Gems says.

In humans, the problem may be part behavioral and part physiological, notes Dr. Gems, who admits that many questions remain unanswered. "One theory is that testosterone raises metabolism, so men burn energy faster and thereby lower their life spans," he says.

The upside is that if all this is true, men probably have a stronger propensity for longevity than women, Dr. Gems says. "If males had the same genetic constitution as women and had all these odds stacked against them, they'd be genetically unfit," he says. It's this stronger innate constitution that also likely explains why men who live to their eighties and nineties are in better shape than women of the same age, Dr. Gems says. "The trick is getting out there," he says.

Preferably with all appendages still attached.

Getting Out of Your Genes

The Lifestyle That Fits

Scientists recently have found a bad bit of DNA floating around in the genetic coding of mankind. If you inherit it from one of your parents, this dangerous DNA can increase your risk for having a heart attack by 50 percent. Inherit it from both your mother and your father, and your risk doubles.

This is just the latest in a slew of findings from geneticists who are reporting that a man's susceptibility to common killers such as heart disease, high blood pressure, and prostate and colon cancer can be passed down to him at birth, putting him in a high-risk category from the moment the cord is cut. This news—coming as it does after a decade of doctors telling us that a healthy lifestyle was all we needed to by-pass most life-threatening conditions—has left many wondering how much control we actually have over our own health.

The answer: a lot. Scientists are investigating these genetic connections not to dole out death sentences but, rather, to show people what may lie down the road so that they can take the proper measures to head it off at the pass. Lifestyle changes can have an enormous impact on de-creasing your risk for diseases, says Dr. Walter M. Bortz II of Stanford University School of Medicine.

Researchers at the Southwest Foundation for Biomedical Research and the University of Texas Health Science Center, both in San Antonio, found that among 1,236 Mexican-Americans who were part of 42 extended families studied, genes accounted for only 15 to 30 percent of various risk factors for heart disease. So in most cases, Dr. Bortz says, our risk for the diseases that commonly kill men is determined by how we live.

All in the Family

Though many hospitals are equipped with Orwellian, high-tech equipment that can read your genetic legacy from a single drop of blood, the easiest way to know what's in your genes is to look at your family tree, says Dr. John J. Mulvihill of the University of Pittsburgh.

"You can definitely see your prominent risk factors in your family history," Dr. Mulvihill says. "And we're learning more all the time. Ten years ago, we didn't think there was any family linkage to prostate cancer. Then people started talking about it and uncovered a strong family connection. The problem is that most men don't know their family history."

Worse, even when they do know, most don't give it a second thought. Of the 58 people interviewed for one study, nearly half of those having family members who suffered from heart disease or cancer did not believe that their family history had any bearing on their own risk. And men were much less likely than women to think that having a family member afflicted with cancer was relevant to their own risk for the disease. Despite their disbelief, studies show clear connections.

In Japan, for in-stance, researchers com-paring 363 people with colorectal cancer with an equal number of people who were cancer-free found that those having one first-degree rela-tive (a parent, sibling, or child) with colorectal cancer had almost twice the risk of developing the disease as those with no family history of colon cancer. In a similar Canadian study, researchers found that 15 percent of 640 men with newly diagnosed cases of prostate cancer had at least one blood relative who also had the disease, while only 5 percent of 639 men who did not have prostate cancer had any family ties to the disease.

And almost nowhere is family history a stronger link than it is for heart disease. As mentioned earlier, just inheriting one tiny bit of faulty DNA from both Mom and Dad can double your risk for developing heart disease.

In the final analysis, we're all likely to be at genetic risk for something, concludes Reed E. Pyeritz, M.D., Ph.D., professor of human genetics, medicine, and pediatrics at Allegheny University of the Health Sciences in Pittsburgh. "I'm fairly convinced that, to some degree, all disease is genetic. So far, the major common diseases to which we've identified genetic links include Alzheimer's disease; arteriosclerosis and all that comes with it, like heart disease, hypertension, and stroke; diabetes; and, of course, most forms of cancer. There's surely more to come."

That's all the bad news. The better news is that studies show these genetic risk factors can be largely offset by making appropriate lifestyle changes or by seeking early medical help in some cases.

What's in Your Hands

Though family history is a strong indicator of the diseases that may be in your future, it is far from the last word, Dr. Pyeritz says. "Two people can have the same high-risk gene mutation, and one will get the

Thunder in Your Genes

If one of your early childhood memories is Dad sawing logs on the La-Z-Boy after a good evening's meal, you are ripe to carry on the tradition whether you care to or not. Like the color of your eyes, snoring can be passed down the gene line.

In one study, researchers from Denmark questioned 3,308 men about their snoring habits, family history of snoring, blood type, and other lifestyle factors. They considered "habitual snorers" men who reported snoring often or always. Among the habitual snorers was a subgroup of men considered to have a more severe form of snoring because they had been relegated to a separate room during nonwaking hours. After analyzing all possible connections, the factors they found that most strongly separated the most serious snorers from habitual snorers were age and—you guessed it—family history. The researchers also found family history to be the factor most strongly separating habitual snorers from nonsnorers.

While snoring is certainly a nuisance for anyone who shares your bed, or even your house, it can also be downright dangerous. Snoring can be a symptom of sleep apnea, a condition in which breathing actually stops during sleep, causing oxygen deprivation and, over time, leading to high blood pressure and an enlarged heart.

Though the researchers didn't offer any solutions for getting out of your snoring genes, Edmund Pribitkin, M.D., an otolaryngologist at Thomas Jefferson University Hospital in Philadelphia, advises perpetual snorers to try sleeping on their sides rather than their backs, to steer clear of late-night alcoholic drinks or sleeping pills (since both can bring on some noisy Zzzs), and to lose weight and exercise.

disease and the other will not. It's hard to know one way or another when we're talking about one gene among 99,999 other genes that also have some influence," he says.

But the greatest influence is exerted by the lifestyle choices—some small, some large—that you make every day: whether you smoke, how much you drink, what you eat, whether you exercise.

The following are some tips that experts offer for taking your health into your own hands.

Know your tree. "You should retrieve all the information you can about your family history and what diseases run in your gene line," Dr. Mulvihill says. "When it comes to fighting disease, knowledge is power. When we know what we're up against, we can keep on the watch for it and do all we can to prevent it. A good example of how helpful this can be is the skin cancer called melanoma.

"If you've inherited a mole pattern on your skin that contributes to melanoma, you're not going to change that," Dr. Mulvihill continues. "But before we started identifying people with this risk pattern, the death rate was much higher. Now that we know what to look for, some of these folks may still get the disease. But we catch it in stage one, so people don't die from it."

Keep a running tab. Knowing you're at risk does you little good if you don't bother watching for signs of disease. That's why Dr. Ken Goldberg of the Male Health Institute recommends keeping tabs on yourself, including performing a monthly testicular self-exam, a skin exam for changes in moles or unusual markings, a quick check of your glands for swelling, a heart-rate check, and a scan for lumps around your chest. If you have high blood pressure or have had a high blood pres-

---

A History Lesson

Often there is no better way to know what diseases you need to be on the alert for than to take a quick look up your family tree and see which ailments have been hanging around for a generation or two. It's also important that your family doctor know your family's medical history, says Dr. Reed E. Pyeritz of Allegheny University of the Health Sciences.

"Your doctor should be especially aware of conditions that are 'special' within your family—meaning any common disorders that occur with high frequency and diseases that occur at particularly young ages," Dr. Pyeritz says.

The following worksheet, from *How Men Can Live As Long As Women* by Dr. Ken Goldberg of the Male Health Institute, can help.

Your Family History

Definitions: Immediate family includes father, mother, grandparents, brothers, and sisters. Second-degree relatives are uncles, aunts, and cousins.

1. What have your immediate family members died from, and at what age?

_____

_____

---

sure reading, you should also have your blood pressure checked monthly. And if you have a family history of or are at risk for diabetes, you should have your blood glucose measured monthly as well, says Dr. Goldberg. If your blood pressure and blood glucose are normal, you need have them checked only once a year, he adds. (See Medical Testing on page 62.)

Recognize your inherited habits. Bad habits often can run as strongly down the family lines as bad genes, says Dr. James

2. What have your second-degree relatives died from, and at what age?

_____

_____

3. What medical problems do or did they have?

_____

_____

4. What medications do or did they take?

_____

_____

5. What habits, good and bad, do or did they have?

_____

_____

6. What kind of surgeries or other hospitalizations have they had?

_____

_____

7. What kind of exposures to toxins have they had at work or elsewhere?

_____

_____

common environmental factors that trigger that disease and avoiding them is your best line of defense, Dr. Mulvihill says.

People who are at high genetic risk for colon cancer may be able to lower their risk for polyps by following a low-fat, high-fiber diet because they're staying away from known triggers, Dr. Mulvihill says.

Likewise, diabetes is often a case of genetic tendency meeting an environmental trigger, says Dr. Mulvihill. Genes that predispose many people to adult-onset diabetes were probably survival genes for our ancestors to help them store energy during prolonged periods of near-starvation. Today, when these genes are combined with the typical sedentary Western lifestyle and high caloric intake, we end up with obesity, insulin resistance, and adult-onset diabetes. The answer again is to control what you can, Dr. Mulvihill says. And that's how you live. It's well-known that avoiding high-fat, high-sugar fare is a good way not only to keep off excess pounds but also to avoid adult-onset diabetes.

Finally, when it comes to beating your odds for heart attack, there's still nothing better than giving your lifestyle a good spring cleaning, says Dr. Ichiro Kawachi of the Harvard School of Public Health.

"Things like not smoking cigarettes, eating less fat and junk food, eating more fruits and vegetables, exercising, and relieving stress are a whole lot more important than worrying about your genes," Dr. Kawachi says.

Genes or no genes, the incidences of heart disease and stroke have decreased markedly during the past 30 years because people have been taking their health into their own hands, says Dr. Pyeritz.

Enstrom of the University of California, Los Angeles.

Take an inventory of your habits, Dr. Enstrom says. Do you smoke? Do you exercise? Do you sleep enough? How much do you drink? Do you eat too much? While these things are important for all of us, they're particularly important for folks who have a history in their family of poor health, he says.

Don't pull that trigger. Once you've tracked down your disease profile, learning the

The Great Mystery

What Happens When You Die?

When his number was up, Timothy Leary, the king of the counterculture, embraced dying as one of the greatest journeys man can make. Just after midnight on May 31, 1996, surrounded by close friends, Leary went into the great beyond. His last words were, "Why not? . . . Yeah."

Leary had long expressed interest in being put into a deep freeze via cryonics after his death, with the hope of being "reanimated" sometime in a science-fiction future. He reportedly had a change of heart a few weeks before his actual departure because he had "other plans" for his after-death. Instead, his remains were boosted into orbit aboard a Pegasus rocket.

There's not much anyone really knows about what happens when we die—try though we may to find out what's really behind the curtain before we actually have to step backstage ourselves. From attending our first day of Catholic school to picking up our first prophecy by Kahlil Gibran, most of us have given at least some chunk of thought to the great beyond. And most of us believe that something—whether it's coming back here for another try or lying in the big eternal bed made from our earthly deeds— awaits us in the afterlife. But since most folks don't come back once they go, we're forced to rely on faith rather than facts about the life hereafter.

Even things that should be cut-and-dried about death and dying—things like when death actually occurs in the body—aren't as simple as you'd

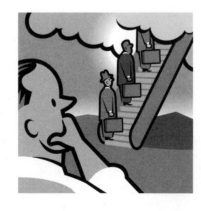

think. Though scientists have a pretty good idea about how we die, attitudes about when a person is officially dead are not only radically different among various cultures but also have even changed and continue to change within our own.

When Are You Dead?

Historically, people have been shockingly bad at determining when their fellow human beings were dead. Things got so bad that in 1896 a group fearful of waking up in their final resting place founded the Association for the Prevention of Premature Burial. Earlier in Russia, savvy salesfolk were hawking coffins with a system of flags and bells to summon help should you find yourself buried alive.

The truth is that, until relatively recently, the onset of putrefaction was the only truly reliable sign of death. "Otherwise, you've been considered dead when the medical folks say you're dead," explains Cyril H. Wecht, M.D., forensic pathologist and coroner in Allegheny County, Pennsylvania. "While that hasn't changed, thankfully, we've developed better ways of determining death these days."

A couple of centuries ago, long before the magic of medical technology, just having fainting spells could send you to your grave, recounts Kenneth V. Iserson, M.D., professor of surgery at the University of Arizona College of Medicine and director of the Arizona bioethics program, both in Tucson, and author of *Death to Dust*. "Many diseases like syncope (a condition that causes people to faint or suddenly lose consciousness) and typhoid could easily be mistaken for death in those times."

As recently as 1926, medical texts were advising doctors to look for "signs of life," using uncertain techniques such as placing an ice-cold mirror close to the person's mouth to check for breathing, and cutting an artery to see if the person would still bleed.

They eventually discovered more advanced ways to determine death, based largely on the idea that when your heart stopped, you were dead, Dr. Wecht says. "But then CPR (cardiopulmonary resuscitation) began reviving people whose hearts had stopped. And in 1968, a South African doctor further complicated things by performing the first heart transplant," he says. That's when the folks at Harvard Medical School declared and promoted the idea of "brain death criteria." When your brain has stopped working, that's absolutely the end, explains Dr. Wecht.

Today, doctors have several surefire methods for determining when the brain dies, ranging from the simple (testing the person's ability to breathe on his own and blinking in response to touching the cornea) to the high-tech (hooking the person to an electroencephalograph machine to monitor brain activity, electrocardiograph to measure the heart's electrical activity, and nuclear medicine brain scans). "No one has ever failed all these tests and still regained consciousness," Dr. Iserson says.

Cause of Death

If you've ever wondered how, precisely, people die, we can tell you the one place you should not look for answers: television. On TV, sometimes folks die an agonizing death from the slightest case of sniffles. Other times, the helicopter slams into the bridge and the whole A-Team emerges unscathed.

"It's hard to answer the question of whether death itself hurts because nobody really knows," Dr. Iserson says. There can be pain and discomfort at the initial onset of a fatal event, especially with trauma or where a heart attack or a terminal illness is involved. "But it's not likely that the final moments are very painful since the brain is shutting down. In fact, some dying processes, like drowning, can actually be quite peaceful,"

says Dr. Iserson, a near-drowning victim himself. Here's a quick look at how we die.

The big three. The three top causes of death—heart disease, cancer, and stroke—are also the easiest to understand. They cause death by shutting down vital organs. Most heart attacks occur because the heart is not getting enough oxygen through plaque-constricted coronary arteries. The heart stops, and the lights go out. Stroke is similar but occurs when the brain, not the heart, fails to get enough blood (which is why some doctors now refer to stroke as brain attack). And cancer kills by impairing the functions of the organs it invades.

Bang! You're dead. Fatal events such as car crashes, falling from high places, or being shot cause trauma. More than half of the time, death in trauma cases is actually the result of injury to the heart, a major blood vessel, the brain, or the spinal cord, which causes blood loss and shock or massive injury to the brain or other vital organs. "That's why the Safety Council folks are so adamant about people wearing seat belts, helmets, and other protective gear," says Dr. Wecht. "Often if you can protect your head, you can stay alive."

Bleeding to death. We tend to think of bleeding as something we do on the outside. But internal organs such as the spleen, liver, and lungs are like miniature blood banks. Rupturing such organs can cause massive internal bleeding, which takes precious amounts of blood out of circulation. A quick loss of 40 to 50 percent of your blood, which is approximately five to six pints in a 170-pound man or four to five pints in a 130-pound woman, is enough to cause coma and death. When too much blood is taken out of circulation, the heart speeds up to try to compensate for the loss. But once the pressure and volume get too low, the person falls into a coma, and the oxygen-deprived heart stops.

From gallows to swallows. Finally, there's asphyxiation. One sure way to put your heart to rest and your brain to sleep for good is to cut off your air supply. When you can't breathe, whether a chicken bone is lodged in your throat or cement shoes tied to your feet haul you down to drown, you experience asphyxia. During asphyxia, the pulse quickens, the blood pressure rises, and the amount of carbon dioxide in your blood shoots up due to the lack of new air coming in, or of old air being expelled. In a few minutes, the heartbeat becomes irregular from lack of oxygen and then stops.

Though death accounts are predictably grim, experts say that your final moments, if you are dying from a chronic, natural illness, probably aren't all that bad—even if they aren't exactly pretty. "In many cases, it's just a slip out of consciousness," Dr. Iserson says.

Going into the Great Beyond

From biblical times to today, people who have skirted the edges of death occasionally come back to report a world beyond that is, well, beyond imagination. Such events are called near-death experiences, or NDEs for short. With modern resuscitation technology reviving people from further into the dying process than ever before, an increasing number of people return to report visionary experiences.

You've likely heard some of these accounts. Typically, NDE survivors will report floating out of their bodies and actually watching their own resuscitation efforts. They usually recall a long dark tunnel with an astonishing light at the end that they liken to the presence of God. Often they hear music or see people from their past. Then they are sucked back into their bodies as they are successfully resuscitated, sometimes angry at the medical team for saving them.

Classic Comebacks

Our fear of death and the great beyond has fueled a seemingly endless supply of myths and lore, not to mention bad B-movies. Here are a few of our favorites.

Count on "the count." **With Tom Cruise's portrayal of the Vampire Lestat in *Interview with the Vampire*, the world marked nearly 1,000 years of vampire lore. Popularized in the late 1800s with the publication of Bram Stoker's novel *Dracula*, the notion of vampires first appeared in 1047, when someone referred to a Russian prince as "Upir Lichy" or wicked vampire. Vampire hysteria ran rampant from 1600 through the 1700s. Things got so bad in Romania that they developed "automatic vampire-piercing devices"—sharpened stakes driven into the grave so that if the body tried to leave, the vampire would be pierced instantly.**

Essentially, vampires are thought to be folks who have died before their time, often violently, who have come back to kill their family and friends. Telltale signs of vampires are needle-sharp incisors used to suck blood from their prey. A wooden stake through the heart, cutting off the head, or burning the body to ashes are the best-known ways to bring one down for good.

Do the zombie. **Countless cult classics like *Night of the Living Dead* show once-dead and buried folks clawing their way from their earthly tombs and oozing into nearby neighborhoods to wreak havoc among once-happy, unsus-**

Not surprising, controversy abounds surrounding the science of NDEs. Some researchers in the field estimate that up to nine million adults in this country have had such life-altering NDEs. Some people look to faith for an explanation. Others speculate that they are biological events—the result of psychological defenses or of a brain-chemical mix that

pecting citizens. Though nobody can say for certain where the concept of so-called zombies came from, it's one we clearly dread—and one that may be more reality-based than you think.

Reportedly, Haitians schooled in the science of voodoo could administer a fish poison known as tetrodotoxin that would induce a state just inches from death. The victim would then be buried and, provided the voodoo maker had administered just the right dose, could later be "resurrected" to terrorize the living.

Tell it to your mummy. Ancient Egyptians believed that they were "magically resuscitated" after they died. To help the dead along, they would first embalm the corpse to mummify it. Then they'd bury it in an elaborate tomb, equipped with furnishings and toilet facilities so that the mummy could live comfortably once he came back to life. Somewhere along the way, people began to worry that maybe the mummy would wake up not in the Egyptian afterlife but in his tomb, mad as hell, and with a hankering to take his anger out on the living.

Today, we're less nervous about that possibility but just as fascinated with mummies. More than 100,000 people a year travel to Kampehl, Germany, to view the remains of Christian Friedrich von Kahlbutz, a seventeenth-century count who was found naturally mummified in his crypt.

According to Bruce Greyson, M.D., professor of psychiatric medicine at the University of Virginia School of Medicine in Charlottesville, it makes perfect sense that not everyone who is resuscitated reports a near-death experience. "Many people who come close to death suffer a small amount of brain damage," says Dr. Greyson. "Even brief periods of unconsciousness can leave them with amnesia for events. So it's not surprising that so few remember NDEs."

As for the argument that NDEs are no more than a dying brain's response to lack of oxygen, Dr. Greyson says that's nonsense. "Oxygen deprivation produces agitation, confusion, and idiosyncratic hallucinations, totally unlike the calmness, exceptional clarity of thought, and consistent visions of the near-death experience," he says. "And the few studies that have actually measured blood oxygen levels in near-death situations have shown no correlation between oxygen deprivation and near-death experiences." Furthermore, NDEs also often include memories of events—such as details from the resuscitation efforts—that the near-death experiencer could not possibly have seen, Dr. Greyson says.

No matter which side of the argument you weigh in on, it's hard to deny the long-standing belief that there is something beyond this mortal life here on Earth. The ancient Egyptians believed so passionately that they would be "magically resuscitated" after death that they built lavish tombs for the dead to contain all the items they would need in the afterlife (what do you think the Pyramids are?). Today, Islamic as well as Christian people believe that God will ultimately raise the dead for an everlasting life. Buddhists and Hindus, too, believe in a cycle of life, death, and rebirth.

occurs during death to cause a hallucinatory effect. Other medical experts are skeptical that NDEs exist at all. "I have been resuscitating people as an emergency physician for many years, and I have yet to see a person have a near-death experience," contends Dr. Iserson. "Most often, they remember nothing at all."

Death with Dignity

Don't Fear the Funeral Director

If you're the average 40-ish man holding this book in his hands, by the time you're ready to call it a night in a permanent kind of way, it may cost $12,000 to $15,000 to give you a respectable funeral and lay your body to rest.

That's right. What it would cost to buy that Jeep Wrangler you've been eyeing up at Marty's Big Trucks is close to what your loved ones will have to pay for your final departure somewhere down the road. And as if that wasn't bad enough, statistics show that you could wrack up bills nearing $100,000 during your final days in the hospital, which, unless fully covered by insurance, can leave an enormous hole in the money you leave behind for your family.

And you thought your kids' college tuition costs were going to send you to an early grave?

No doubt about it, there's a better way. While the main focus of this book is on how to live longer and enjoy every minute of it, the simple fact is that we're all going to die eventually. And like living, we'd prefer to do it on our own terms where possible. For many men today, that means dying without lingering, assisted by machines, far beyond the point of enjoying life anymore. It means leaving their family financially secure and with lasting memories of a life well-lived.

Making Wanted Advances

There was a time when doctors were applauded for

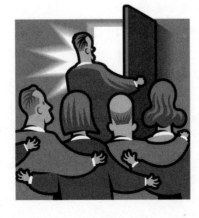

doing everything humanly possible to keep us alive. Then medical technology blasted off like the starship *Enterprise* into realms where no man had gone before, allowing gravely ill people with no hope for recovery to be sustained on machines almost indefinitely.

That's a fate that many of us have come to fear more than death itself. "Most people want to die with dignity," says Ron Aldrich, president and chief executive officer of Advance Directives International, a business designed to educate people about living wills and other so-called advance directives. "And being allowed to waste away on life-support machines is not what they have in mind."

You can make sure that your wishes are carried out in two simple ways—a living will and a durable health-care power of attorney, says Aldrich. The one you choose depends upon your circumstances.

Living will. A living will is a document that lets you put in writing which medical treatments you want and which you do not want at the end of your life. Contrary to misperceptions, that does not mean that you will be denied emergency care that could save your life.

"People often ask, 'Will 911 respond to my call once I have a living will?' " says Steven A. Litz, an attorney in Allentown, Pennsylvania, who practices in the areas of elder law and estate planning. "The answer is absolutely. You'll always receive emergency medical care and be transported to the hospital." Living wills come into play only when you have a condition that will cause death no matter what the doctors do. You're in a coma. Or you're in what doctors call a persistent vegetative state—your body will work, but your brain will not. Living wills are concerned only with processes that prolong the dying process, as respirators and feeding tubes often do.

Even then, the doctors will pull out the living will only if you can no longer speak for yourself.

Durable health-care power of attorney. This document allows you to put someone you trust in charge of your health care in case you aren't able to make decisions yourself. "This is a good document to have in cases where you're incapacitated, but you're far from dead, as is often the case with people who have Alzheimer's disease or brain damage," Aldrich says. Durable health-care powers of attorney cover a wide array of health-care issues, including admitting or discharging you to a nursing home or hospital, accepting or denying treatments, donating your organs, ordering an autopsy, and even making arrangements should you die. "It's very important that this person know exactly how you want to be treated," Aldrich says. "So you need to tell them—in writing." There are legal forms you can fill out that make your wishes clear in a wide array of medical situations. You can also choose more than one agent so that one can act as a backup.

Don't know where to start? There are numerous places that provide advance-directive services. Try the Department of Aging in your county, your local hospital, or a specialized advance-directive firm. Or just see your lawyer, says Aldrich.

"None of these options is very difficult or expensive to arrange," Litz says. "A living will can cost as little as $25 to prepare by a lawyer." The following are some more tips to help you get the most from your advance directive.

Check your church. Most religions support advance directives, says Aldrich, who frequently fields this question. Some religions, however, have reservations about such documents, particularly living wills. To be certain, he

---

Words to Die By

There's no more dignified way to leave this world than to use your last breath to deliver a one-liner that'll go down in history. Here are some of the best.

"I only regret that I have but one life to lose for my country."
—Nathan Hale (1755–1776), American Revolutionary spy; speech before his execution, September 22, 1776

"I'm bored with it all."
—Winston Churchill (1874–1965), British Prime Minister; the great speech-maker's final words before slipping into a coma and dying nine days later on January 24, 1965

"Et tu, Brute fili."
—Julius Caesar (100–44 B.C.), Roman dictator; last words to his assassin and supposed ally

"Goodbye, kid. Hurry back."
—Humphrey Bogart (1899–1957), American actor; last words to Lauren Bacall as she left the room for a moment on January 14, 1957

"Go on, get out—last words are for fools who haven't said enough."
—Karl Marx (1818–1883), German Socialist; last words to his housekeeper upon her urgings for his last words so that she could write them down for posterity

---

recommends that you check with your minister, priest, rabbi, or spiritual leader if that's a concern for you.

Talk to your doc. It's a good idea to tell your doctor about your advance directive not only so that he knows that this document exists should it become necessary but also because some doctors may not agree with your wishes. Doctors do not have to honor advance directives if they conflict with their own religious or spiritual beliefs. If your doctor has a conflict, he should be able to direct you to a health-care provider who will honor your wishes.

Spread the word. Once you've signed a living will, Aldrich recommends giving copies to family members, close friends, clergy, your doctor, or anyone else who might be called upon to carry out your wishes or to help make end-of-life decisions for you.

Keep it current. If you have a sudden change of heart about your directive, be sure to change your form as well as your mind, Aldrich advises. "Advance directives are living documents that can be altered, but you have to tell everyone who has a copy, especially your doctor, so that they can tear up the old one and replace it with a current form," he says.

Prearranging Your Final Arrangements

Every day for the final three weeks of his life, the ailing King Charles V of Germany and Spain demanded to have a funeral service and to be carried around in the coffin that would eventually be used for his burial. After all, funerals are for the living, right?

Though you won't likely be able to persuade friends and family to go that extra mile during your last days, one of the perks of prearranging your funeral is that you can have things the way you'd like them.

"Most men who come in to prearrange their funerals are cost-motivated," says John H. Brubaker, a funeral director in Catasauqua, Pennsylvania. "But then some find that they like being able to personalize the service."

Brubaker has seen his share of funerals "American-style." "People are buried with all sorts of things," he says. "Golf clubs, cigars in their pockets—you name it." The music is another place where folks like to add a personal touch. "One man loved Elvis, and that's what they played," recalls Brubaker. "Another was a member of a polka band, so we had some polka music playing softly in the background. It's a celebration of a life well-lived."

The potential to have it your way aside, the biggest benefit of prearranging your funeral is saving your wife and kids the enormous burden and expense at a time when they'll already be carrying a heavy load.

When you consider the professional services such as burial preparation, transportation, and facilities as well as the casket, vault, church expenses, flowers, and other funeral merchandise, the average cost of a funeral and burial is between $5,000 and $6,000 plus the cost for the grave site, Brubaker says. And prices may vary depending on where in the country you live (and die). Even a simple cremation service runs between $1,000 and $4,000. And that's without having your ashes spread over Wrigley Field.

"What we do is take the exact figure of what a funeral would cost today and invest it in an interest-bearing account—like a CD (certificate of deposit), a master trust fund, or life insurance—which makes up for inflation," explains Brubaker. "Generally, there's more money in the fund at the time of death than is needed. In that case, the family gets the difference. In the rare event that there isn't enough money, we pay the difference." Not all companies work this way, Brubaker adds, so make sure that you find out whether yours does before signing on the dotted line.

The best part is that once it's done, it's done, says Brubaker. "Once you make the arrangements, it's all taken care of. And you and your family never have to worry about it again."

That said, with the rise in funeral prearrangements has come a rise in people getting ripped off, says Brubaker. Keep the following in mind when you're prearranging those final touches.

Get it itemized. In 1678, the funeral bill for a Hartford, Connecticut, man who had drowned included a pint of liquor for the men who dived for him; a quart for those who brought him home, and more than eight gallons of wine and a barrel of cider for the funeral.

Not what you had in mind? Then get an itemized bill. It'll keep you from paying for what you don't want—or get.

Fill in the family. The idea of prearranging your funeral is to give your family peace of mind. So once you've made arrangements, let everyone close to you know that you've made your plans and outline what they are, Brubaker says. Better yet, include them in the arrangement-making. It sounds a tad morbid, but if you're already planning your funeral, it might not hurt to ask their feelings on the matter. After all, funerals are as much for the living as they are for the dead.

Update as necessary. Playing *(I Can't Get No) Satisfaction* during your wake may have seemed like a good idea 10 years ago, but now you're thinking more along the lines of Beethoven's Ninth Symphony. No problem. You can rearrange your prearrangements as you see fit, says Brubaker. Just let the funeral director in charge know, and make sure that the change is put in writing. "It's also a good idea to let your family know about any changes you make," Brubaker adds.

Getting Your Affairs in Order

You've appointed your wife durable power of attorney. You've ordered a polished oak casket that shines like your first baseball bat. And you've footed the bill for the whole shebang, saving your loved ones enough headache and expense to qualify you (if posthumously) as Husband and Dad of the Year. You're done and never have to think about it again, right? Almost.

Here are just a few more things to add to your "Dying with Dignity Checklist," according to our experts.

Make a will. Many families have a story of an irreparable rift caused by bickering over an estate. "Sadly, this happens even when there's not a great deal to fight over," Litz says.

That's why everyone over age 18, rich or poor, should have a will, he says.

"Without one, it's a race to the courthouse to determine who ends up as administrator of your estate," Litz says. "Then the registrar of wills ends up choosing, which can be a legal nightmare. It is essential to have a will if you have children under 18 years of age. In a will, a guardian is named to take care of your children and a trustee to take care of your estate for the benefit of your children." You should also name someone you trust as the executor of the will to file with the court and see that your wishes are carried out. "A will is a simple way to be sure that your money and possessions go exactly where you want them to go," concludes Litz. "A lawyer can help you make all the arrangements generally at costs less than $150."

Keep good records. You should write down and gather up everything you think the executor of your estate will need, suggests Brubaker. Include your biographical information, which is essentially the information needed to fill out a death certificate and to write an obituary; your financial information, including your Social Security number, your most recent income tax returns and W-2's, last Social Security check (if applicable), marriage certificate, spouse's Social Security number, and any military records; the location of your will; your insurance policies; children's names, addresses, and telephone numbers; bank accounts and securities; safe-deposit boxes; benefit entitlements; and other important documents.

Know your benefits. "Too many people have no idea what benefits they're entitled to," says Brubaker, who is often the first person to tell them. He recommends that people find out what benefits they're entitled to through the places they've worked, Social Security, and the armed forces, and make a list of them. Most of these benefits are not automatically paid when you die. Your family needs to apply for them.

The Quest for Immortality

Show That You Were Here

Legend has it that young James J. Kilroy was like any other working stiff in the 1940s, loading freight ships day in and day out. Then one day he had a flash of how he could be just a little bit more. Chunk of white chalk in hand, he scrawled, "Kilroy was here" on a mother lode of crates full of blue jeans waiting to sail to harbors across the globe. When that slogan—generally accompanied by a face peeking over a wall—started popping up around the country, including such inaccessible places as the Statue of Liberty's torch, the once-anonymous Kilroy achieved immortality.

"We all have a little Kilroy in us," says Dr. Walter M. Bortz II of Stanford University School of Medicine. "We want to leave a legacy to show we were here. We have an inherent want for immortality. And that's a healthy thing."

Live Forever

There are a whole lot better ways to have your name live on than etching your John Hancock on a bathroom wall. Many can actually leave the world a better place. Others are just plain fun. So strap on some of these suggestions and rocket into eternity.

Sign a donor card. "The absolute best way for anyone to live on after their death is to make an organ, tissue, or whole-body dona-

tion," says Dr. Kenneth V. Iserson of the University of Arizona College of Medicine. "There is a dearth of organ donors in this country, and the need for transplantable organs and tissues is enormous—and getting bigger."

The number of people who have died while waiting for available organs has increased more than 2½ times during the past eight years, according to the United Network for Organ Sharing in Richmond, Virginia. And every 16 minutes, a new person is added to the national transplant waiting list. Donor families consistently report that they feel their loved one is living on in someone else through their organ donation. Considering that about 25 different organs and tissues are transplantable, that's a lot of immortality.

You can get a donor card from a local or regional organ or tissue bank, or you can fill out a donor card when you renew your driver's license. Even if you have the sticker on your driver's license, doctors most likely will still check with your family before donating your organs.

Make a carbon copy. Though God knows it shouldn't be your only motivation, one of the benefits of having children is that you leave behind a living legacy. Your kids will not only carry on your tale about that 36-inch walleye you reeled in last summer but also pass on the only part of you that is truly immortal—your genes.

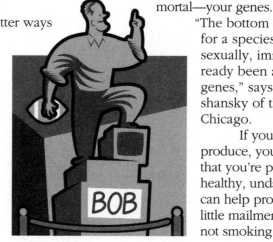

"The bottom line in life is that for a species that reproduces sexually, immortality has already been achieved through its genes," says Dr. S. Jay Olshansky of the University of Chicago.

If you should decide to reproduce, you want to be sure that you're passing along healthy, undamaged genes. You can help protect those mighty little mailmen of immortality by not smoking and by getting plenty of vitamin C, say experts. Studies show that nicotine damages sperm and reduces sperm count. Vitamin C, on the other hand, has been shown to protect the little guys from free-radical damage.

Bank your genes. To get the benefits of having a Junior to carry on your genes, without all the 5:00 A.M. feedings and Saturday soccer practices, you might consider making a donation at a sperm bank, where they freeze your sperm for women and couples seeking artificial insemination. You'll get immortalized DNA, no added responsibilities, plus between $35 and $50 in, uh, hard cash for each effort.

Be forewarned, however, that sperm banks can be more discerning than a potential mate. "There's a meticulously involved screening process," says Charles Sims, M.D., co-founder and medical director of the Los Angeles–based California Cryobank, one of the country's largest sperm banks. "Before you can even think about donating sperm at California Cryobank, you must be between the ages of 19 and 39, enrolled in or have graduated from a four-year university, be at least five feet nine inches tall, be of appropriate weight for your height, and know your medical history for three generations back," he says. Only about 8 percent of prospective donors squeak through the sperm bank's gates.

Pass it along. It's a waste to have your prized polka banjo get snapped up by some stranger for $5 at a Grandpa's-no-longer-with-us yard sale. That's what family heirlooms are all about—immortality through sentimentality. By passing a treasured item down the family line, you can be remembered fondly for generations to come.

Freeze!

One of the most dramatic stabs you can take at immortality is putting yourself in a deep freeze after you die, with the hopes that future medical wizards will have the technology to bring you back as good as, if not better than, new.

Here's the drill. You pay to become a member of a cryonics organization, like CryoCare Foundation in Wilmington, Delaware. Then, when you're near death, the cryonics folks dispatch a medical team to wait by your bedside. When an independent medical professional pronounces you legally dead, the cryonics team takes over, submerging you in ice water, replacing your blood with a fluorocarbon similar to antifreeze, and eventually cooling you to –196˚F and sealing you away in a storage vault.

Until when? Nobody knows, but certainly not until medical science can cure cancer, heart disease, or whatever else killed you as well as fix the phenomenal amount of tissue damage that freezing causes. "Currently, that damage cannot be reversed," concedes Ben Best, one of the founding members of the CryoCare Foundation. "But we believe that doctors in the future will be able to. When you consider all the advances medical science has made so far, including cloning, it isn't that far-fetched."

The price: a minimum of $58,500 to freeze just your head (under the assumption that they'll be able to build you a new body later), and $125,000 for your whole body.

An heirloom can be anything from your District IX track-and-field trophy to your Gibson Flying V guitar. Just be sure to put in writing what the item is and what it means to you, and then pass that along with your heirloom so that your great-great-grandson Shmecky doesn't inadvertently toss your family treasure in the circular file. Chances are that your relatives will also appreciate the heirloom that much more if they have a clear understanding of its history and significance.

Make a time capsule. One inexpensive, easy, pretty cool way to immortalize yourself is by making a time capsule, says Paul Hudson, co-founder of the International Time Capsule Society (ITCS) in Atlanta.

Consider including items like copies of birth and marriage certificates, job reviews, pictures, golf scorecards, passports, a copy of the *Sports Illustrated* swimsuit issue, your favorite bowling shirt, compact discs, and anything else you think best represents your place in time.

"The best time capsule container is a safe. But you can use any container with a cool, dry, dark interior," says Hudson. "Then mark a time for it to be opened in, say, 50 or 100 years, and place it in a secure place indoors. Don't bury it outside, though. Thousands of time capsules are lost that way." You can also register your time capsule with the ITCS by writing to Oglethorpe University, 4484 Peachtree Road NE, Atlanta, GA 30319, and they will add it to their database so that there will be an official record of where your time capsule is and when it was created.

Plant a sapling. The planet will always need trees to clean the air, give birds a home, and provide shelter from the cruel sun. So why not give the earth one in your (or someone else's) honor and have folks remember you for it? Sure, you could just stick a tree in your backyard and mount a plaque by it. But to make it a little more official you can contact American Forests Famous and Historic Trees, 8701 Old Kings Road, Jacksonville, FL 32219.

For $35 plus shipping and handling, they

Last Requests

A dying wish, a last request—it's a wonderful way to make your want for immortality known. Though there's no saying that your survivors will honor your wishes after you've moved on, there's no reason that you can't make them—and make them good. Take a cue from Mark Gruenwald, the late Marvel Comics editor. When he died unexpectedly at age 42, the publisher of Marvel Comics reportedly honored his last request to have his ashes mixed with comic book ink. Gruenwald literally became one with the work he loved when that immortal ink was used in a special reprint of "Squadron Supreme," a limited-edition comic that he had written while he was alive.

will send you a tree variety of your choice along with a personalized certificate of authenticity, which includes a space to record who planted the tree, where it was planted, and in whose memory it is dedicated. You also get a lifetime guarantee, so if the tree dies, they'll send you a replacement for only the cost of shipping and handling.

Hitch your wagon to a star. If you're famous enough to be immortalized on the Hollywood Walk of Fame, disregard this entry. If you're not, you can get a star all your own without ever having to get your hands glopped up with cement. And it'll be a real one—guaranteed to last a couple of billion years, or at least longer than you likely will.

For just $49.95 you can have your very own star named after you, complete with a registration certificate, a page showing the celestial address of your star, and a constellation chart to help you find it so that you can show your friends. Just contact the folks at Name a Star, a division of M&M Associates, at P. O. Box 1020, Fort Jones, CA 96032, for more information.

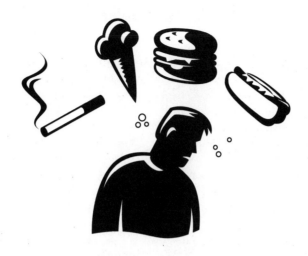

Part Two

The Age Extenders
Arsenal

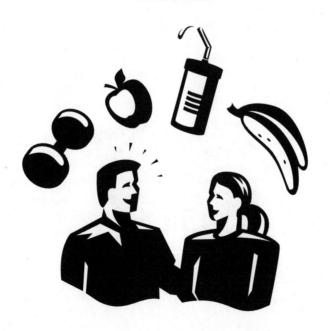

Alcohol

The Spirit of Good Health

There has been very little middle ground when it comes to alcohol. Prophets, poets, and medicine men have been extolling its life-enhancing virtues since biblical times. Yet modern medicine, recognizing its harmful effects on the heart and liver and its tremendous contribution to accidents, has been reluctant to give even the slightest nod of approval to drinking alcohol.

But now, as the evidence mounts in its favor, even the most stoic medical heads are nodding acknowledgment that in moderate amounts—which means no more than two drinks a day—alcohol can actually do a body good. But what's "one drink"? One drink equals 12 ounces of beer, 5 ounces of wine, or 1½ ounces of 80-proof hard liquor.

To Your Heart's Content

It all started with the French. They smoke. They eat cheese and crackers. They practically make butter a food group. Yet somehow they manage to have a death rate from heart disease 2½ times lower than ours. When scientists explored the reason why, they uncorked an answer that surprised everyone—red wine.

Red wine is brimming with stuff called phenolic compounds. These compounds— with $10 names like quercetin, resveratrol, and catechin—give red wine its rich scarlet hue. Though we need more research to understand exactly how they work, scientists believe that these compounds also attack heart disease on two fronts.

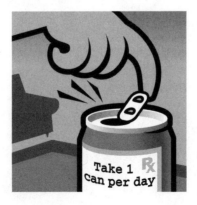

Take 1 ℞
can per day

First, they work similarly to aspirin, keeping the platelets in your bloodstream from sticking together and forming blood clots. Second, they are antioxidants. That means that they help neutralize free radicals, which are unstable oxygen molecules that damage your body's low-density lipoprotein cholesterol and make it more likely to stick to your artery walls, causing them to block and harden, explains Andrew L. Waterhouse, Ph.D., wine chemist and assistant professor in the department of viticulture and enology at the University of California, Davis. "Besides heart disease, free radicals may also contribute to cancer and even aging," Dr. Waterhouse says.

Though wine was the first "adult beverage" scientists said could actually be good for your heart, they've recently given some good news to Guinness-lovers as well. Dark beer can provide protection similar to red wine, and even lighter beer seems to provide mild protection, according to John D. Folts, Ph.D., head of the coronary thrombosis research laboratory at the University of Wisconsin Medical School in Madison and a renowned researcher of a type of phenolic compounds called flavonoids—natural substances which are supposed to lower risk of heart disease. To prove that flavonoids in beer might have some health benefits, Dr. Folts mechanically narrowed the arteries of 16 dogs and gave them drugs to make their blood clot. Then he poured each dog either a Guinness Extra Stout or a light-colored lager made by Heineken. The 11 lucky dogs who got the Guinness had all their clots cleared. Those given the Heineken had their average number of clots reduced from seven to four. Dr. Folts attributes the benefits to the more numerous flavonoids found in dark beer.

There's even a bit of good cheer for those who prefer vodka, white wine, and other drinks that don't contain many dark-colored flavonoids, says Ichiro Kawachi, M.D., Ph.D., associate professor of health and social behavior at the Harvard School of Public Health. Just plain alcohol in small amounts may provide heart protection all its own. A review of several studies on the effects of moderate drinking and heart disease concluded that four found benefits from drinking wine; four found benefits from beer; and four from spirits. "That's because alcohol raises your levels of healthy HDL (high-density lipoprotein) cholesterol," says Dr. Kawachi. The evidence is clear, he says: Moderate drinkers do better than abstainers in decreasing their risks of heart attack.

The Cancer Connection

Though heavy drinkers have higher risks for cancers in areas like the mouth, esophagus, and liver, people who drink less—six or fewer drinks a week—show no increased risk. And those who drink moderately may actually lessen their risk for lung, prostate, and other cancers, say scientists.

Researchers in Chicago found that one particularly potent wine compound, resveratrol, not only fought cancer at several stages but also actually seemed to reverse it. In a similar study, researchers from the University of California, Davis, found that when they fed dehydrated wine solids to mice who had been genetically altered to develop cancer, those who ate the wine feed took approximately 40 percent longer to develop tumors than the mice who didn't eat the wine solids. "The antioxidant properties of the phenolic compounds like catechin and quercetin may play a major role in this cancer prevention," says researcher Susan E. Ebeler, Ph.D., of the University of California, Davis. "But we need more research to know for sure."

Are You Drinking Too Much?

One in 10 people who drink will become an alcoholic. While moderate drinking yields health benefits, problem drinking wrecks lives. If you have trouble with alcohol, you should not drink at all, states the National Council on Alcoholism and Drug Dependence. Check yourself for the following signs that you may or could develop a problem with alcohol.

- *Heredity.* If your mother or father had a drinking problem, your risk is fourfold.
- *Drinking more than two.* The national government and other experts draw the line at two drinks a day for men. Drink more than that and you put yourself at higher risk for developing a problem.
- *High tolerance.* If you drink excessively without really feeling any ill effects, you also may have a drinking problem.
- *Secret drinking.* If you're sneaking drinks, won't talk about your drinking, feel loss of control, or have blackouts, you need help with your drinking.

Living Longer, Living Better

Alcohol doesn't just help against the biggest life-threatening ailments. There is scads of research to show that moderate drinking can ward off other common health problems—the kind that can make life pretty miserable sometimes. Here's a catalog of the conditions you can raise a glass to.

Beating the runs: Diarrhea may not be particularly life-threatening to you, but there's no doubt that it diminishes your quality of life, especially when you've plunked down a couple grand for the vacation of a lifetime and all you've seen is the inside of the international john. Believe it or not, wine may help here, too.

Wine has long been used as a digestive aid across the world. Now researchers know why. When scientists were experimenting with ways to kill some of our most vicious intestinal foes, including *Escherichia coli* and salmonella, they tried dousing them in test tubes with wine, tequila, ethanol, and bismuth salicylate—better known as Pepto-Bismol. Though the bismuth salicylate did okay, wine was the overall winner—killing more than six times as many bacteria as the pink stuff. (The tequila and the ethanol had no effect on the bugs.) And it seems that just six ounces may be enough to do the trick.

Getting unstoned: Kidney stones aren't exactly lethal, but passing one is enough to make any man wish he were dead. You'll be happy to know that a couple of beers a day can keep the kidney stones away, according to Harvard researchers.

After surveying more than 45,000 men intermittently over a six-year period, the researchers found that men who drank two or more beers a day were four times less likely to develop kidney stones than men who didn't drink. Wine was not quite as effective, but it still cut the kidney stone risk in half.

Keeping your wits: Your head may also enjoy a small nightcap, but not in the way you think. You probably already know of alcohol's ability to remove all memory of, say, that drunken line dancing episode. What you don't know is that in much lesser amounts, alcohol may actually boost your memory.

According to a study by researchers in the Netherlands, folks who have a drink or two a day seem to be half as likely to have poor thinking ability as teetotalers. And French researchers found that among 2,273 people older than 65, those who drank 8 to 16 ounces of wine a day were much less likely to develop dementia, which may be an early stage of Alzheimer's disease, than people who drank less or no wine. We need more research to further explain how alcohol works. Luckily, there's no shortage of volunteers for future studies.

Living longer in general: With the combination of all these benefits, it seems that a daily bottle of beer or a glass of wine may actually extend your life.

In a 12-year study of more than 13,000 people, researchers in Denmark found that people who drank a couple of glasses of wine a day lived longer than folks who never touched the stuff because they had lower risks for heart disease and stroke. And in the land Down Under, Australian researchers studying 1,236 men over age 60 found that those who drank reasonable amounts of alcohol regularly—anywhere from one to three drinks a day—lived significantly longer than men who completely abstained. Another study, this time of 490,000 people ages 35 to 69 by the American Cancer Society, concluded that moderate alcohol intake in this age group slightly reduced deaths from all causes.

Rules to the Drinking Game

Finally, an umpteenth reminder: If your local tavern hails you as the reigning champion of Three-Man and Mexican Dice, you likely won't enjoy any of the benefits we've listed here. To get the most out of alcohol, you have to drink responsibly. According to guidelines established by the federal government, here's how.

Don't play averages. You can't save up your one or two drinks a day and have 14 on Friday night instead. You should drink no more than two drinks a day. Don't binge.

Wait until the dinner hour. Lunchtime is not Miller time. Even one drink during the workday slows you down mentally and physically. Save it for when you get home.

Go right on red. Though health benefits of moderate alcohol consumption are associated with all types of alcohol, remember that red wine is the way to go for antioxidant phenolic compounds. Researchers from the University of California, Davis, tested 20 California wines and listed the most phenolic-rich types. Try one of these next time you're out: Merlot and Petite Sirah.

Companionship

"Opening Our Hearts" Is Good Medicine

Medical science has proved that "Only the Lonely" is a more accurate selection than "Only the Good Die Young" if we're trying to pick the true hits on the Grim Reaper's jukebox.

The lonely, the disenfranchised, the disconnected, those who feel their lives have no purpose—studies show that these are the folks at greatest risk for coming down with a bad case of premature death or life-threatening disease, says Dean Ornish, M.D., president and director of the Preventive Medicine Research Institute in Sausalito, California, and author of *Dr. Dean Ornish's Program for Reversing Heart Disease.*

Amazingly, in a study directed by psychologist Sheldon Cohen, Ph.D., professor of psychology at Carnegie Mellon University in Pittsburgh, people with the most diverse types of social contacts and networks were the least likely to be susceptible to a cold virus intentionally squirted up their noses. More on that in a minute.

Why does social interaction seem to have a life-lengthening and health-promoting effect?

"Bottom line: Nobody knows," Dr. Ornish says. What *is* known, he says, is that "it is the quality, not the quantity of relationships" that matters.

That's What Friends Are For

So no one knows for sure why mingling and sharing thoughts and feelings with others

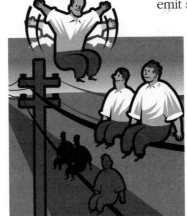

is healing. Theories abound. Dr. Cohen and his research cohorts at Carnegie Mellon believe that having a wide range of social environments is distracting—and that's good. "For example," Dr. Cohen says, "someone whose only social role is worker will find problems at work more distressing than someone who works, has a family, and belongs to social groups."

Whether we call it distress or just stress, it truly is a killer, Dr. Ornish says. Much of his program for heart attack patients is devoted to helping them learn to reduce stressful responses. "We know that when people are under stress, their immune systems are impaired and their cardiovascular system is more prone to heart attacks or sudden cardiac death," he says.

In Dr. Cohen's study that we mentioned earlier, participants' blood levels of norepinephrine and epinephrine were measured regularly. These two hormones are released when we are under acute stress. Dr. Cohen's researchers squirted the common cold virus up the nostrils of all the test participants. Those who became infected were those who had the highest levels of the stress-indicating hormones and were those with the fewest types of social contact.

At this point in medical research, however, it is too early to say that we gain the health effects of positive interaction with others because our brains instruct our glands to exude some protective chemicals—or our brains emit specific electrical impulses—that strengthen our immune systems, Dr. Ornish says.

Dr. Ornish and colleagues have implemented and studied the effects of programs "that increase the sense of connection and community, and we have found that the patients initially think that this is the part of the program that will be least helpful. And yet when they have gone through the program, they find that it is the most powerful and meaningful part." That's because the peer interaction encourages people to stick with positive helpful behaviors, such as healthy diets, ceasing smoking, and other goals the programs set forth for the patients, Dr. Ornish says.

"People who feel lonely and isolated are more likely to smoke, abuse other drugs or alcohol, eat too much, work too hard, or watch too much television as ways of numbing, distracting, or killing the emotional pain that they feel. I think the real epidemic in our society is this emotional or psychological or spiritual heart disease—this sense of loneliness, isolation, and alienation that's so common when people feel that sense of disconnection," says Dr. Ornish. People in the throes of that epidemic are more likely to engage in behaviors that increase their risk of premature death or disease, he says.

So how does one get connected? First, says Dr. Ornish, realize that there is a difference between being alone and being lonely.

"It's not how many people you call every week or how many people live in your household," says Dr. Ornish. "It's not so much the number of social contacts you have but the perception of whether you feel loved and cared for and nurtured by them. Someone could be alone by choice—in a monastery, for example—and they can also feel that sense of interconnection with something spiritual.

"It doesn't necessarily have to be another person," adds Dr. Ornish. "Some studies show that even having a plant to take care of, or a pet, prolongs life. Anything that takes us outside of the belief that we are separate and only separate, I think, is healing. The word *healing* even comes from the root 'to make whole.' "

Feeling Better

In order to establish meaningful contact with other humans, you have to learn how to talk—openly. Learn how to communicate in ways that let others hear you better. A key, says Dr. Ornish, is to practice expressing feelings rather than thoughts. Feelings connect; thoughts—particularly judgmental ones—isolate us, he says. Here are some of Dr. Ornish's communication tips.

• Express a thought—"I think you're wrong," for instance—and your listener may feel attacked and argumentative. Express a feeling, though—"I feel sad about what you said," for instance—and the listener is more likely to hear you, Dr. Ornish says.

• Express feelings and you make indisputably true statements. No one can argue about how you feel. How you feel is how you feel.

• Express feelings and you exhibit a bit of vulnerability that people generally recognize and respond to in kind, raising the level of the communication.

• Feelings—that is, emotions—are more effective than thoughts in influencing people.

It is just as important to express negative feelings as positive ones, Dr. Ornish says. Just learn to express them as feelings, not as judgments or attacks. Add the words *I feel* to your vocabulary. One caution, though: Dr. Ornish says that if you add the word *that* after an *I feel*, you probably are not truly expressing a feeling but, rather, a thought.

One way to encourage more expressions of feelings rather than thoughts is to rid your language of the phrases "You should," "I think," "You ought," "You never," and "You always." Instead, add the phrase, "I want."

We communicate more intimately when we acknowledge what we hear other people saying to us, making it clear that we really listened and really heard what they said and making sure that we understand their meaning, Dr. Ornish notes. Try it and you'll see that people warm to you as they feel more understood. And you will warm to them, too, because you will be focusing on their feelings and expressions, rather than paying more attention to what you're going to say next.

Getting a Connection

Once you've mastered the art of talking and listening more effectively, there are other steps you can take to widen and deepen your social circle, Dr. Ornish says. Here are the actions he recommends.

Practice altruism, forgiveness, and compassion. It's in your own selfish best interest, says Dr. Ornish. A major 12-year study showed that men who never do volunteer work are 2½ times more likely to die young than those who volunteer at least once weekly.

Compassion and forgiveness, says Dr. Ornish, simply are healing emotions. Help others in ways that you feel comfortable doing so—and never because you feel forced to, he advises.

Share secrets. Every man needs at least one other person in the world with whom he can feel free to be himself completely, to confide in. Find people and groups with which you feel comfortable letting down your hair.

Be a joiner. Clubs, church, study groups, support groups, any ongoing positive social interaction in which we have an opportunity to develop a sense of community encourages us to be self-disclosing and is healing and helpful, Dr. Ornish says.

Meet your "higher self." Develop your sense of communion and connectedness

---

The Science of Living Together

Scientific studies have rather consistently demonstrated that companionship contributes to good health. The quality of relationships also is a factor, found Xinhua Steve Ren, Ph.D., assistant professor at the Boston University School of Public Health and research health scientist with the Center for Health Quality, Outcome, and Economic Research of the Veterans Affairs Medical Center in Bedford, Massachusetts. Here are some of his other findings.

• Separation and divorce can actually improve health—but only in cases where there were serious ongoing marital problems. Separation and divorce are most detrimental to health when the marriage had no prior serious problems and the crisis arose with the sudden discovery of infidelity.

• Being separated is more injurious to health than divorce. The separated were more than 2 times as likely to consider themselves in poor health than were married folks, while divorced people were about 1.3 times more likely to think themselves in ill health.

• The quality of a relationship—whether marriage or cohabitation—affects the participants' health. Those in unhappy relationships are at higher health risk than those who are in happy relationships and, surprisingly, even than those who are divorced.

• Compared to married people, the unmarried tend to have higher death rates from all causes, have higher levels of stress, and use more health services.

---

with God or a higher sense of being, advises Dr. Ornish. "On one level we're all separate, you and I," he says. "On another level, we're part of something larger that connects us. . . . Having that spiritual vision, that double vision, being able to see both the unity and the diversity, is a very powerful healing experience for many people."

Breathing Techniques

Take It All In

Unless you've had lessons, chances are that you don't know how to breathe. And that's trouble, says breath researcher and psychologist Gay Hendricks, Ph.D., who has taught Olympic athletes and thousands of other people how to breathe at his Hendricks Institute in Santa Barbara, California.

Dr. Hendricks conducted experiments and reviewed more than 300 scientific studies of "breathwork" while researching his popular book *Conscious Breathing*. He is convinced that most of us could use a few breathing lessons. Here's why.

Breathing is how we rid most toxins, like carbon dioxide, from our bodies and how we cleanse and oxygenate our blood and every cell, says Dr. Hendricks. The remaining wastes are discharged through urine, sweat, and defecation. If we aren't breathing right, other purification systems—such as our kidneys—get overworked.

But, Dr. Hendricks says, "there is one universal breathing problem: the tendency to hold your belly muscles too tense so that you can't get a deep breath down into the center of your body." Instead most of us breathe from the top of our lungs. Here's the problem with that. "Less than 1/10 liter of blood per minute flows through the top of the lungs; 2/3 liter per minute flows through the middle of the lungs, and more than a liter flows through the bottom," says Dr. Hendricks.

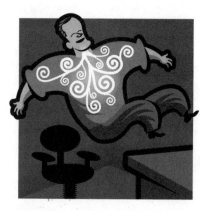

The chest breather constantly discharges too much carbon dioxide and takes in too little oxygen through short, shallow breaths. The imbalance forces the heart to work unauthorized overtime, and that raises the blood pressure.

Health Benefits

Correct, deep, belly breathing, says Dr. Hendricks, has been shown to:

- Melt tension. It counters the shallow tight breaths produced by the instinctive fight-or-flight response that we find ourselves kicked into frequently.
- Clarify and focus the mind.
- Increase energy and endurance.
- Clear unpleasant emotions. Two or three big breaths at the onset of an injurious emotion such as fear, anxiety, or depression are often enough to move it out of the body.
- Help manage pain. (This is why it is taught in natural childbirth classes.) Do not hold your breath when in pain or anticipating pain. Instead, breathe—calmly, deeply.
- Improve athletic performance.
- Significantly lower blood pressure.

Deep breathing and breathing in general help in treating many modern-day maladies.

"Breathing exercises are a major emphasis of the yoga classes I teach in Hawaii," says Arthur Brownstein, M.D., medical director of the Princeville Medical Clinic and clinical instructor of medicine at the University of Hawaii John A. Burns School of Medicine in Honolulu.

Breathing exercises are also a major component of the stress-management program taught to heart patients during the highly touted programs conducted by the Preventive Medicine Research Institute in Sausalito, California.

Doing It Right

The following are the basics of Breathing 101, as taught by Dr. Hendricks as well as Barbara Lang, who teaches Yogic breathing at the Duke University Center for Living in Durham, North Carolina, in an intensive medically supervised program for people with heart problems and other degenerative diseases.

Get past tense. Tense your abdomen. Relax your abdomen. Tense your abdomen. Relax your abdomen. Do this maybe a dozen times, until you are well aware of how a relaxed abdomen feels.

Give yourself a hand. Put your hand on your abdomen. Breathe slowly, comfortably, deeply enough to make your hand rise with each inhalation and fall with each exhalation.

Go for ribs. Keep breathing slowly, comfortably and into your belly. If you are truly breathing correctly, you will feel your rib cage expand to the side with each inhalation.

Move your spine. "Babies can lie in a crib all day without getting a backache because they move their spines with each breath," says Dr. Hendricks. "We tend to hold ourselves more stiffly as we age." With each in-breath, let your spine move away from the chair back (if you're sitting) or away from the floor (if you're lying on your back). On each out-breath, let it flatten against the chair or floor.

That's your basic, healthy breathing. To remember to do it, associate the term *breathe* with normal everyday activities such as standing, sitting, or turning, says Larry J.

Catch Your Breath

We take about 20,000 breaths each day. For a healthy man that should translate into 12 to 14 breaths per minute, says breath researcher and psychologist Dr. Gay Hendricks. Catch yourself breathing normally and calculate your per-minute rate. If it is higher than that, your health is in jeopardy and you should make deep, comfortable, slower breathing a priority, Dr. Hendricks says.

Much of the "breathwork" taught by experts today is drawn from ancient Oriental spiritual teachings. Many of the health claims for ancient Taoist, Hindu, and Yogic breathing exercises have been substantiated in the laboratory. One such exercise, alternate nostril breathing, is a proven tension-tamer and mental energizer, Dr. Hendricks says. Here's how he teaches it.

Close off one nostril with the index finger of your dominant hand and breathe out and then in through the open nostril, slowly, gently, fully. Then close off the other nostril, still using your dominant index finger, and breathe out and then in through the open nostril. Keep your belly muscles relaxed and breathe comfortably, slowly in and out of your abdomen. Put your attention on the sensations of the breath leaving your nose and the breath returning. Alternate like this for two minutes, and then switch to the index finger of your nondominant hand and continue for two minutes. Switch back to your dominant hand for one more minute, and then rest for a minute with your hands in your lap. Just don't try it while you have a runny nose.

Feldman, Ph.D., director of the Pain and Stress Rehabilitation Center in New Castle, Delaware. Then, he says, taking healthy, deep breaths at intervals throughout your day will be as natural as, well, breathing.

Fitness

It's Your Best Weapon

Maybe somewhere deep inside you lurks that crazy thought we all have in our more irrational moments. To wit: Can't this whole disease-threat thing just go away? Can't a society that put men on the moon and all of Merle Haggard's work on CD come up with some kind of high-tech anti-illness potion so that we can go on about our business?

Hang on, we have one for you. Behold our magic pill, guaranteed to significantly reduce your risk of disease. It's fun to take. It makes you feel good. It's 100 percent natural. It's cheap and available.

Okay, we exaggerate a tad—but only by the smallest of tads. It's not guaranteed (nothing is in medicine). It's not a pill. And it's not magic. But fitness through exercise is a proven disease risk–reducer. Go down the list of killers and exercise combats most of them.

In short, a regular fitness program should be the cornerstone of your antidisease strategy, experts say.

Working Out Disease

"The numbers clearly show that people who are physically active have less disease," says Kerry Stewart, Ed.D., a clinical exercise physiologist and director of cardiac rehabilitation and prevention at Johns Hopkins Bayview Medical Center in Baltimore. "Particularly heart disease."

Since heart disease is the number one killer of Americans, that's no insignificant piece of

information. Exercise works its wonders directly and indirectly. Directly, according to Dr. Stewart, it improves things like heart function and body metabolism. Indirectly, it works on the risk factors of disease. For example, exercise lowers high blood pressure, decreases your percentage of body fat, and improves your ratio of "good" cholesterol to "bad" cholesterol. All of those things are major factors in heart disease.

But fitness fights more than just heart disease. It's the treatment of choice for diabetes as well as your best bet to avoid it. And only recently has exercise's cancer-fighting value come to light, most notably (for men) as a risk-reducer for colon and prostate cancer.

Exercise not only keeps you alive but also keeps your life worth living. "Most of what people think of as 'growing older' isn't," says Walter M. Bortz II, M.D., clinical associate professor of medicine at Stanford University School of Medicine and author of *Dare to Be 100.* "It's disuse. They don't understand the power of exercise."

The Aerobic Answer

The concepts of "health" and "Grateful Dead concerts" don't often appear in the same sentence. But those enthusiastic souls who used to shake their whatevers nonstop while the Dead played 1½ hours straight (without tuning up once) were faithfully, if unwittingly, engaged in a noble health pursuit—aerobic exercise.

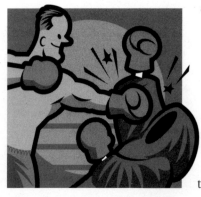

Jane Fonda–style aerobic dance classes may have publicly appropriated the word, but the truth is that any activity that jacks your heart rate up for an extended period of time is aerobic exercise. That means running, cycling, swimming, rowing, skiing, in-line skating, or anything else that gets you huffing and puffing enough to feel it but not so much that you can't keep it up.

All those good things that exercise does to help you avoid heart disease come mostly from aerobic work. That's eminently logical when you bear in mind that what aerobic exercise essentially does is strengthen your heart (hey, it's a muscle, too) and improve your lung capacity, thus helping the flow of oxygen through your bloodstream.

Aerobic exercise is also the principal player in diabetes prevention. "Regular aerobic-type exercise will allow you to metabolize your blood sugar without requiring as much insulin," says Ben Hurley, Ph.D., director of the Exercise Science Laboratory at the University of Maryland's College of Health and Human Performance in College Park. "That's important for both heart disease and diabetes prevention. And the research is very consistent." If you want to take advantage of aerobic exercise's health benefits, here's all you need to do.

Do as you please. The kind of aerobic exercise that works best is whatever kind you'll do. So your wisest choice, according to physical therapist Mark Taranta, director of the Physical Therapy Practice in Philadelphia, is to go with what you like. "Do something you're familiar with or enjoyed doing in the past," he advises. "Don't go out and buy a big piece of equipment like a treadmill if you've never tried it before. You might hate it."

Get that heart rate up. Any exercise expert will tell you that to reap the full benefits of aerobic exercise, you have to do it hard enough. Sorry, golf won't cut it. (No, not even if you carry your clubs and take 130 strokes to finish.) The aerobic effect doesn't kick in until your heart's beating at 70 percent of its maximum rate.

Your maximum rate per minute, by the way, is 220 minus your age. So if you're 40, you want to have your heart beating at 70 percent of 180 beats per minute while you're exercising. (We'll do the math for you, this time only—it's 126 beats per minute.) Check your pulse by putting two fingers to the side of your neck and counting the beats for 10 seconds; multiply that by six, Taranta says.

And keep it up. Once you get your pulse up to 70 percent of your maximum, keep it there for at least 20 minutes. While you're working your way up to that magic 20-minute mark, remember that accumulating the time over a 24-hour period (say, three seven-minute sessions on the stationary bike) will provide almost the same benefits.

Stick with it. If you get your aerobic workout three to five times a week, you'll be amazed at how quickly the positive changes kick in. But you'll be just as amazed at how fast they fade if you start backsliding. "If you don't keep at it, you lose it," Dr. Bortz warns. "The gains and losses are very transient. If you want to translate them into genuine health benefits, you have to do it regularly."

Be reasonable. Assuming that your fitness goal is achieving overall health rather than medaling in the Olympics, it makes more sense to enjoy your exercise sessions than to turn them into torture tests. Yes, there are the minimum requirements we've mentioned, but you don't have to go much beyond them. "It doesn't take a whole lot to maintain your cardiovascular fitness," says Tom Baechle, Ed.D., chairman of the exercise science department at Creighton University in Omaha, Nebraska. "We've gotten away from the killing-yourself mode. You can get it done in 20 minutes a day, three times a week, at a reasonable intensity."

Strengthening: Your Defense

Lifting weights makes you stronger because your muscles will adapt to the extra stress you're putting on them. So you look better and you feel better. You're also healthier, in ways that a lot of people don't normally associate with muscle building.

For example, strength training builds lean muscle mass, which helps to burn more calories. In doing so, it helps to burn fat, which, of course, helps to maintain an appropriate body weight. And trained muscles metabolize glucose much better and lower your insulin resistance. That helps prevent diabetes.

Where strength training really does its job is making you feel more alive. Think about how much dedicated gym rats like to talk about how great they feel. (Some of them, you may have noticed, talk about it a little too much.) Then think about how much other men talk about how lousy they feel as the years go by. Strength training can turn that gym-rat attitude into an ageproof lust for life.

"If you don't want to lose a lot of your muscle power as you get past 40 or 50, strength training can have a big effect," Taranta says. "Without it, you won't be able to do things as well, so your activity level will decrease. This can lead to heart problems, cholesterol problems, hypertension—all of that." Here's how to get the best benefits from strength training.

Shock your system. Lifting weights once in a while when you're in the mood won't get the job done. "You have to shock your muscular system on a regular basis or else muscles will lose their strength," Dr. Baechle says. How often is that? Well, you need to give your muscles a day off after working them with weights, but you shouldn't let them rest more than three days before "shocking" them again, according to Dr. Baechle. "Two days a week will work," he says. "Monday and Thursday or Tuesday and Friday are fairly common systems, but three times a week (for example, Monday, Wednesday, and Friday) is a little better."

Work the major muscles. Those would be your chest, back, shoulders, legs, abdomen, and arms. Some movements with

Off the Couch

When you haven't been off the couch since high school, starting a lifelong fitness program can seem a daunting task. Take it one step at a time, says Douglas Lentz, a certified strength and conditioning specialist and director of fitness and wellness at Results Therapy and Fitness in Chambersburg, Pennsylvania. The following phases make up one painless approach to getting started. Each phase can last a week or more, depending on your chosen pace.

1. *You're climbing off the couch.* "You have to walk before you run," Lentz says. He means it literally. Start by taking a 10-minute walk, three days a week. Sure, there's very minimal aerobic effect yet, but you're introducing your body and brain to a new world. Pick a consistent time for your walk. "If you usually come home and watch television before dinner, walk first and *then* watch television," Lentz says. Start stretching right away. For now, do it at the end of your walk, stretching just your hamstrings and calves, some of the muscles you use while walking.

2. *You're moving away from the couch.* Take your walk up to 15 minutes. Add 5 minutes a week until you hit 20 or 30 minutes, says Lentz. Take your stretching up to five days a week. Add a stretch a week to your routine.

3. *You're starting to forget about the couch.* Boost your walking pace to "brisk." You're on your way to getting your heart rate up to an aerobic-benefiting level. Throw in some strength training, Lentz says.

weights work the entire group; others pick out individual muscles, such as your biceps. "Try to do one exercise for each major muscle group to get a balanced effect," Dr. Baechle advises.

Hit your number. For general health purposes, repeating each exercise 12 to 15 times without stopping is the ideal, according to Dr. Baechle. "That seems to be a number where you can really concentrate on the technique in-

Nothing fancy. Get used to the idea of moving weight around. Do it at home twice a week on the days you don't walk. There's a lot you can do without weights—pushups and crunches are just a couple examples. But buy a pair of weight-adjustable dumbbells to expand your options, Lentz suggests.

4. *You've covered the couch with plastic.* **Jack up the aerobic pace by doing intervals. "If you've been walking briskly for 20 minutes, you may not be able to just start jogging 20 minutes all at once," says Mark Taranta of the Physical Therapy Practice. "So walk for 3 minutes and jog for 3 minutes, walk, jog, walk, jog." Move your strength show to a more organized venue. That means joining a gym, or investing in enough home equipment to work all your major body parts. Taranta suggests keeping your start-up routine simple—one set per major body part, 12 to 15 repetitions, two days a week.**

5. *You gave the couch to Goodwill.* **You're at or near exercise commitment. Start cross-training by shifting your aerobic work from jogging to something else, like a little bike work or swimming to keep things interesting. Keep the interval-training idea alive with whatever activity you choose, working your way up to a steady, challenging (but not exhausting) aerobic pace. Include more body parts (that is, biceps, triceps, calves) in your strength routine, adding a little weight to each exercise as it becomes easy, Taranta says.**

Welcome to fitness.

volved, on the breathing and rhythm, and on range of motion, without being so concerned about how much weight you're lifting," he says.

Learn to fail. The amount of weight you lift varies with the exercise, of course, but the rule of thumb is that the last time through the movement—in this case, say, the 15th repetition—should be the last you could possibly do. That, in weight room talk, is called working to failure, a case where failure is a good thing. Start light. If making it to 15 repetitions is too easy, add weight. If you can't make it to 12, lighten up, says Dr. Baechle.

Do it once and for all. When you finish your 15 repetitions of any exercise, you've done one set of that exercise. If you rest and do it 15 more times, you've done two sets. How many sets should you do? That question starts arguments across the great schism in the church of iron about the relative benefits of multiple sets over a single set. But there's fairly solid agreement that for the beginner interested in general health there's no need for time-consuming extra sets. "One set's enough when you're starting out," Dr. Baechle says. "But for continued improvement, try to increase the number of sets and weight loads as you get stronger."

Get organized. There's a reason that you see those guys walking around the gym making notes between exercises. They're keeping track of what they did and how much they did of it. Catch-as-catch-can workouts are better than nothing, but you need a set routine in order to chart and make progress. "Your body really needs to know what you're expecting of it," Dr. Baechle says. "When you keep changing the exercises, it compromises the muscles' ability to adapt and become stronger. Staying with the same routine for about a month provides an ideal opportunity for muscles to adapt to training."

Besides, there's something encouraging about being able to quantify your progress. "Part of the fun of training is recording the results of your workout," Dr. Baechle says. "It's reinforcing to be able to look back and see how much weight you are using—that is, how much stronger you are."

Living on Flex Time

Men don't stretch. And for good reason: They hate it.

"Stretching's just not fun," says Janet Sobel, a physical therapist and clinical specialist at National Rehab Hospital/Suburban Regional Rehab in Chevy Chase, Maryland. "The results aren't visible. No muscles bulge. And you don't look cool doing it."

But stretching is a joint-saver, according to Sobel, as well as a circulation-promoter, a performance-enhancer, and an injury-preventer. All of those things are important for disease prevention. "Stretching doesn't directly decrease the likelihood of disease," Sobel says. "But by enabling you to exercise without injury, it enables you to do what you need to do to minimize your disease risk."

Here's how to ride the stretch limousine to better health.

Stretch daily (or almost). "Stretching should be like brushing your teeth," says Barbara Sanders, Ph.D., chairman of the physical therapy department at Southwest Texas State University in San Marcos. "It should be part of your daily routine." Since we're talking about only a few minutes to do a handful of stretches that require no equipment, you'll probably find seven days a week doable and even enjoyable. But five is an acceptable minimum, Sobel says. "You're not going to see results if you do it every other day," she says. "But if you do it five days a week, it will pay off."

Hold the stretch, but not your breath. To get the big benefits, you should hold each stretch for 20 to 30 seconds and repeat two or three times, Sobel says. And hold it still—*no bouncing*. At first you'll notice a temptation to hold your breath as you hold the stretch. Resist it. "Breathing is very important," Sobel says. "If you don't breathe, you're going to tighten up and it will hurt. That's counterproductive."

Stretch for as long as it takes. And that's not very long. The only requirement is to work all the major body areas. "A basic stretch routine will be six to eight stretches," Sobel says. Three repetitions of six stretches at 20 seconds each is six minutes. You spend more time than that looking for your bathrobe in the morning.

Just do what you can. What's the most annoying moment in those stretching classes at your health club? How about when the instructor tells you not to worry if you can't go "all the way" in some stretch that looks like it was invented by one of those contortionists in Chinese circuses? All the way? You can't even begin it.

Don't even try, Sobel advises. "Get as close as you can until you feel a comfortable pull, but not pain," she says. "Be attentive to your body's signals. Each person has his own genetic design, and you want to achieve your own potential, not someone else's. Ultimately, you'll get there."

Putting It All Together

"If you want to optimize your health and well-being in all categories, then it's helpful to do cardiovascular exercise as well as strength training and flexibility," Dr. Hurley says.

So how do you put it all together?

Fix your schedule. Compared to keeping your wife, mother, and kids happy, scheduling in your three exercise modes should be simple. For general health, a 3-2-5 plan should work, says Ed Burke, Ph.D., vice president of the National Strength and Conditioning Association in Colorado Springs and co-author of *Getting in Shape*. Put your two strength-training days between your three aerobic days, and stretch on all five. You're still at a half-hour a day, and you have the weekends off.

Try the combo special. You can even cut down your days from five to three by doing aerobics and strength training at the same time. "You can actually get an aerobic workout by doing weight training.," Taranta says. "Go from station to station or exercise to exercise without taking long breaks so that you maintain a high heart rate."

Warm your muscles. There are lots of good reasons to warm up before working out. For one thing, warming up puts your brain in sync with your muscles, making them ready to be called upon to work hard. "And common sense tells us that warmed-up muscles are probably going to be less likely to be injured," Dr. Baechle says. "Plus we know that warmed-up muscles are able to pick up and use oxygen more efficiently."

When exercise experts talk about warming up, they mean it. Do something to raise the temperature of the muscles you're going to be using. In weight training, for example, that could mean duplicating the motion of the exercise at very low weight. "Just pick the exercise you're going to do and use about half the load," Dr. Baechle says. "If you're warming up for an activity, make it specific for that activity. Using one-half of the training load in an exercise is a great way to make it specific."

Stretch out your workout. "Most of us who are 35-plus grew up thinking that warming up was stretching," Sobel says. "It's almost the opposite. You want to warm your body up and *then* do your stretching. Warming up involves increasing the body's temperature and heart rate through low-level aerobic, full-body activity."

In fact, a good time for you to stretch is *after* you've done your aerobic or weight workout. "If you cool down by stretching, you don't get that after-exercise soreness and you get more of the stretching benefits," says Sobel.

Move It On Up

It's one of life's more satisfying certainties. At some point, you're going to hit a plateau in your exercise program. You want more challenge, more fitness, more health benefits. How do you get more?

Here's a sampler of available intensifiers that will actually decrease your exercise time.

Be efficient. Examine your habits a little. You probably spend an inordinate amount of gym time staring in the mirror or resting or flirting. All those things have their place in life, but you'll be better off lifting weights. "Take fewer breaks in between your sets," suggests Mark Taranta of the Physical Therapy Practice. "Decrease your rest time. Increase your efficiency."

Fail more successfully. Instead of adding sets or repetitions, add enough weight so that you reach failure. Sure, you were supposedly doing that all along, but were you? Honestly? "Keep your repetitions at 12 to 15, but find a way to do it so that you really can't do more than 15," Taranta says.

Slow it down. Go ahead and reduce your lifting days. Or your sets. Or your repetitions. Or even the weight load. But here's the trade-off: "Do each repetition a lot more slowly," Taranta says. "Take two minutes to do a set instead of 30 seconds." The slow-moving approach works the muscles much more intensely than the quicker version, according to Taranta. "You're recruiting more muscle fibers," he says. "When some fatigue and give up, others take over."

Jack up the pace. Timesaving intensity applies to your aerobic endeavors as well. "On occasion, do it just twice a week but with an increased heart rate," says Taranta. "Go much harder for three-minute intervals."

Food

Cultivating a Taste for Life

Doctors tracked 11,000 health-conscious people for 17 years, watching, you might say, every bite they put into their mouths.

These researchers at the Imperial Cancer Research Fund in Oxford, England, and the Department of Public Health and Policy in London and the University of Wales in Cardiff recorded each person's diet, illnesses, and deaths, when they occurred over the 17 years.

Two groups of people turned out to be the healthiest—that is, they had the lowest rates of debilitating diseases and were the least likely to die young. The winners were the apple-a-day folks—those who ate some fruit daily—and the garden-grazers—those who ate fresh salad daily. Salad-eating in particular was linked to a 26 percent lower rate of death from heart disease.

While this study was conducted in Great Britain, its findings apply to those of us here in the colonies as well. Want to spend more time on the planet? Then spend more time thinking about what you put on your plate.

Take Control

We have more control over the grub we grab than about any other aspect of our lives. How we stuff our faces controls, to a great extent, the quality of our lives. It significantly influences our health, vitality, and longevity, notes Carla Wolper, R.D., a nutritionist at the Obesity Research Center at St. Luke's–Roosevelt Hospital and the Center for Women's Health at Columbia-Presbyterian Hospital, both in New York City. Every cell in our bodies depends upon the proper supply of nutrients. We get our nutrients from the foods we eat.

Of course, you already know that. You know that you should eat right.

You know that experts recommend eating from five to nine servings a day of fruits and vegetables. But we know that if you're a typical guy, you aren't getting five to nine servings a day of fruits and vegetables.

We're not here to yell at you about that (well, not too much, anyway). But we would like to reason with you or, at least, to give you some reasons to make sure that you're eating a balanced diet—one that includes plenty of fruits and vegetables.

For starters, the doctors and scientists we spoke with emphasized over and over that plant life contains a whole arsenal of goodies that are known, without a doubt, to guard against all sorts of nasties—from premature aging to cancer. Among the most powerful weapons are:

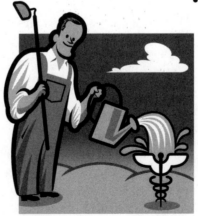

- Plant pigments: The stuff that causes plants to have color turns out to be chock-full of a veritable rainbow of beneficial vitamins and enzymes that our bodies crave.
- Phytochemicals: These chemicals act as a plant's natural defense system—its natural pesticides and disease-fighters. Some of these chemicals help us ward off the scourges that attack us, too.
- Plant estrogens: These are plant hormones, sometimes referred to as phytogens, that seem to enhance and balance hormonal activity in our own bodies. Estrogen? you ask. Aren't we getting a bit girlish here? Not really. See, we need some of these so-called female hormones to cool down some of the male hormones—like the one that causes prostate cancer, for instance.

The Pyramid: A Monument to Good Eating

The four-tiered "food pyramid" is our government's best guess of how we should eat to be healthy, based on current science. It seems to work pretty well, says Melanie Polk, R.D., director of nutrition education for the American Institute for Cancer Research in Washington, D.C. So just what does the pyramid tell us to eat?

Be
frugal
with the fats.
Fats, junk foods,
oils . . . use them spar-
ingly. Do some dairy. Two
to three servings of milk, yogurt, or cheese. That's 1 cup milk or
yogurt per serving; about 1½ ounces hard
cheese. Be miserly with meat. This may surprise you, but you need only two to three servings
of meat, poultry, fish, dry beans, eggs, or nuts a day. A
serving is ½ cup cooked beans, or one egg, or 2 to 3 ounces
cooked, lean meat, poultry, fish, or soy-based burger. Feast on fruits
and vegetables. That's the next-biggest tier. Three to five servings of
vegetables daily and two to four servings of fruit. A serving is a cup of raw
leafy vegetables, or a half-cup of other vegetables. A medium apple is a serving.
So is a medium peach or orange. Go for the grains. That's bread, cereal, rice, pasta.
We should eat more from that group than any other—6 to 11 servings daily. Note
that serving sizes are usually smaller than we think. Read the nutrition information on the
package. One slice of bread is a serving. One ounce of cold cereal is a serving. One ounce.

• Flavonoids: The tasty stuff that gives fruits and vegetables their flavors turns out to be medicine in our bodies.

Then there's the other stuff, like the assorted enzymes, vitamins, minerals, and fibers that we get from regularly eating a wholesome variety of vegetables and fruits. Many of these plant constituents act as antioxidants. That is,

they help protect our cells from getting burned and deteriorated from too much oxygen and other destructive atoms showing up in the wrong place at the wrong time. Antioxidants slow the aging and dying process at the cellular level.

While it is certain that the healing compounds in plants work together when we eat a variety of them, often it is less clear how well they work alone. The research is still young. So the recommendation for now, Wolper says, is to mix it up. Go for variety. Still, there are at least a few superfoods for which the evidence is so strong that it would be foolish to ignore.

Blue-Plate Superstars

Don't eat the following foods to the exclusion of all others, says Edward Giovannucci, M.D., Sc.D., assistant professor of medicine at Harvard Medical School. But these are superfoods that you should include on your shopping list each week and find ways to work into your meals because they increase immunity, build healthy hearts and strong bones, and defend against cancers, arthritis, diabetes, and other debilitating and even deadly diseases.

Bring on the sauce. Tomato sauce, especially when cooked in even the tiniest bit of olive oil, seems to guard against both colon and prostate cancers. Some evidence suggests that it may protect against cancers of the stomach and the esophagus as well. Plus this special sauce may even contribute to agility as we age.

You should have no problem getting your fill of this mighty medicine; tomato sauce works its way into everything from chili to Spanish rice.

The hot nutrient here is lycopene, a substance found in plants that may prevent cancer from occurring by mopping up free radicals. Free radicals are highly reactive compounds that could damage DNA and cause mutations, which could cause cancerous cells to grow.

Lycopene may be twice as potent a cancer-fighter as old-faithful beta-carotene, says Dr. Giovannucci. Tomatoes, both raw and cooked, also contain other antioxidants as well.

Why cook tomatoes in olive oil in these days when all we hear is *fat-free, fat-free*? In experiments, people eating tomato sauce cooked in olive oil got roughly 10 times more lycopene into their systems than did people drinking processed tomato juice, reported Dr. Giovannucci.

Dr. Giovannucci led a five-year study of 47,849 men that found that the guys who ate the most cooked tomato products were the ones with the lowest risk of prostate cancer. Need we say more?

Bag the broccoli. Yeah, we know, it hasn't won any presidential medals. But broccoli is fabulously full of immune system–building vitamin C and features a fistful of the phytochemicals thought to fight cancer. Plus there's a variety of healthy ways to stomach it—steamed, stir-fried, blanched, baked, and raw—even chilled with yogurt dip.

The amount of broccoli you need to eat to prevent disease hasn't been quantified, but broccoli should be among the variety of vegetables you eat, says Walter C. Willett, M.D., Dr. P.H., chairman of the department of nutrition at the Harvard School of Public Health.

Keep cans of kidneys in the cupboard. Kidney beans boast the highest, healthiest fiber mix of any member of the legume family—almost 6 grams per ½-cup serving. They are especially high in heart-protecting folate, too.

Of the fiber, 2.8 grams is cholesterol-lowering, blood glucose–controlling soluble fiber. Kidney beans are associated with a lower risk of heart disease and stroke and protection from colon cancer, says James W. Anderson, M.D., professor of medicine and clinical nutrition at the University of Kentucky College of Medicine in Lexington.

Beans also contain potent antioxidants known as polyphenolics. In test-tube studies, polyphenolics worked better than vitamin C in keeping fat in the blood from oxidizing—the first step in the formation of artery-clogging sludge. Human research is under way, Dr. Anderson says.

If that's not enough, all beans—kidneys and otherwise—are such good medicine that doctors prescribe them to diabetics (along with other high-fiber, complex carbohydrates) because the foods are digested slowly, which helps maintain low blood sugar and normalize insulin responses.

How much do you need to eat to lower cholesterol and provide the other health benefits? Aim for 1½ cups cooked beans daily, Dr. Anderson says.

Believe this fish story. Some fish have a good type of fat called omega-3 fatty acids, and salmon is one of the richer sources of that element. Our bodies use omega-3 fatty acids to make hormonelike substances called eicosanoids, which help regulate processes such as inflammation, blood clotting, and constriction of blood vessels.

Omega-3's appear to assure the orderly inflow of calcium, sodium, and other charged particles into each heart cell, which helps ensure a nice, steady, strong *thump-bump, thump-bump.*

And talk about capable: Fish like salmon, anchovies, and herring, which are all rich in omega-3's, reel in one of the shadiest characters implicated in rheumatoid arthritis inflammation, leukotriene B$_4$. Scientists can measure a significant drop in leukotriene when fish oil is added to the diet.

Omega-3's don't stop there. They also soothe the effects of Crohn's disease (a serious inflammation of the small intestine), may lessen your sweetheart's severe menstrual cramping, and are thought to help stave off depression.

Need more convincing of this fishy health benefactor? One study showed that people who ate the equivalent of just one serving of salmon weekly had half the risk of cardiac arrest as those who ate no omega-3's.

How much, how often? A single 3-ounce serving of baked salmon provides 10 times the amount of omega-3's the typical American gets in a week. Eat at least one serving weekly, experts say.

Tofu you, too. So it sounds a bit like an invective. Too many of us have shunned it as though it were. But this simple, palatable, easy-to-use, and oh-so-versatile soybean derivative is nothing short of a superfood when it comes to our health.

Cultivating a taste for tofu is easy; it can be added to just about anything without changing the taste. Tofu is mild and light-bodied and represents "one of our very best food choices," Dr. Anderson says.

What can you do with tofu? Blend it in a shake or smoothie. Crumble it on a salad. Chuck chunks into soups, stews, chili, marinara sauce. Slice it for a sandwich to replace cheese. Blend it into dips, dressings, custards, puddings. Slip it into stir-fries.

The potential health benefits of soy are sweeping, says Dr. Anderson. Topping the list: major heart protection. Add to that preliminary but encouraging studies suggesting reversal of osteoporosis, and other studies suggesting reduction in the risk of kidney disease and a lower risk of prostate and colon cancers. You begin to see why Dr. Anderson is *soy* excited.

Researchers haven't determined precisely how soy manages its heart-healing magic, but they're thinking that compounds in soy might function as antioxidants.

In addition, emerging research suggests that isoflavones (another plant version of estrogen) in soybeans may actually repair damaged, sluggish blood vessels, restoring their youthful flexibility—something that's important for healthy blood flow, says Dr. Anderson.

The isoflavones' estrogen-like and estrogen-altering activities may be key to the reductions in risks of prostate and breast cancers. These activities may also be why the isoflavones are credited with preserving bone and actually promoting new bone mass. Isoflavones are also known kidney-protectors.

How much should you eat? It depends on what you want. For general health, Dr. Anderson recommends 30 to 40 milligrams of isoflavones per day. (A ½-cup serving of tofu has 35 milligrams of isoflavones, 1 cup regular soy milk has 30 milligrams, and 2 tablespoons roasted soy butter has 17 milligrams.) To tap tofu's help in reversing heart disease and osteoporosis, Dr. Anderson recommends that you triple your daily dose.

Herbs

The World's Oldest Medicines

Weeds, seeds, stems, leaves, roots, flowers—these are the stuff manly medicine is made from. Really.

For example, there's a palm seed that relieves prostate enlargement as well as or better than prescription drugs and with fewer side effects. In your spice rack, there's a seasoning that will lower cholesterol, lower blood pressure, fight minor bacterial infections, and help guard against cancer. Chewing certain roots just plain makes you feel more vibrant. It's true. What's more, about a quarter of modern prescription medicines in North America are derived or synthesized from natural plant remedies just like the ones we've mentioned above—herbal remedies that have been used, in some cases, for thousands of years.

As you'll learn, herbs can help you live longer, better. We think you should know about them. We are not in any way encouraging you to self-diagnose and self-treat any potentially life-threatening illness. Far from that. But we do believe that an informed man should be aware of his options, including the availability of natural healing compounds that often are effective in guarding against common ailments that attack men. You can find these herbs at your nearest health food store. Many are available in drugstores and groceries. Some may even be growing in your own backyard.

The Healing Herbs

Just what are herbs good for? Here's a list of ailments and complaints men face that herbs have been shown to help.

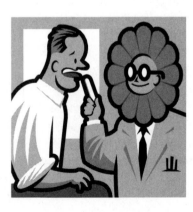

Cutting cholesterol, fighting infections. If you want to do both, garlic is your herb. Eating about a clove per day ought to do it, recommends Varro E. Tyler, Ph.D., dean emeritus of Purdue University School of Pharmacy and Pharmacal Sciences in West Lafayette, Indiana, and distinguished professor emeritus of pharmacognosy (natural pharmaceuticals).

Garlic kills many bacteria, including those that cause ear infections. It reduces cholesterol and keeps blood from clumping and sticking to artery walls, thus avoiding the deadly narrowing of the arteries that can lead to high blood pressure and heart attacks.

Garlic gets its power from a natural antimicrobial ingredient called allicin (pronounced like the girl's name Allison), which is formed when the garlic is chewed or crushed. So if you're going to take your garlic raw, you need to chew it, says Dr. Tyler. Of course, taking garlic that way will get you your allicin, but in the process you may lose your Allison. Dr. Tyler recommends getting your garlic the odorless way—through a coated tablet or capsule. Make sure that the label says it yields between 2,500 and 5,000 milligrams of allicin per dose.

Reversing liver damage. Taking lots of prescription medication over the years, drinking too much alcohol, breathing or ingesting too many pollutants of any sort—all of the above gets processed by the liver. Take in too much of this stuff and the liver can wear out or get damaged. An herb known as milk thistle seems to guard the liver and even help reverse some damage, says Dr. Tyler. The active ingredient here is silymarin. In Europe, doctors have been able to effectively counter otherwise often deadly mushroom poisoning by injecting a standardized form of silymarin into patients. An effective formulation of milk thistle herb should state on the label that it contains 80 to 85 percent silymarin, says

Dr. Tyler. Follow the dosage instructions on the labels.

One milk thistle no-no: Don't down a handful of capsules because you're heading to a party and planning to get smashed, Dr. Tyler says. Taken as an herb, milk thistle is a gentle liver healer, not a poisoning preventive or liver protector.

Protecting against aging.
Sometimes it seems like everybody's *anti* this or *anti* that. Well, that holds true for some herbal remedies, too. Grape seed, for example, is *anti*oxidant. Oxidation is basically the body's equivalent of rust, at the cellular level. It tears down, weakens, and ultimately kills cells that make up our skin and tissues—a process associated with aging and degenerative diseases. Antioxidants, which are found mainly in fruits and vegetables, help counter the cellular wear and tear. How much grape seed should you use? Follow the instructions on the label, says Dr. Tyler.

Ending constipation, reducing cholesterol, guarding against colon cancer. All you have to do is drink slime. That's right. Nice, slimy psyllium in water. Take it flavored or unflavored. Take it as raw husks (which you'll find at the health food store) or as ground-up seeds like those contained in the commercial preparation called Metamucil (which you'll find in the supermarket, along with less-expensive generic versions). Use psyllium daily, says Dr. Tyler, with water and other liquids. *Lots* of liquid—that's key. This bulking fiber, used daily or more often, gently pushes wastes through the intestinal tract. "It acts like a giant sponge going through the gut, swabbing it out. And it tends to remove carcinogens before they can have much effect," Dr. Tyler

Be Careful Playing Doctor

Even chimpanzees do it. Man has used herbs as medicines for at least 5,000 years, and monkeys may have preceded us. We don't know. We do know that they take the bitter herb aspilia to get rid of internal parasites. They don't eat this for fun. They wince as they swallow it, and they swallow it without chewing.

Maybe too many of us swallow without chewing the belief that herbs can't do us any harm, that they are safe because they are natural. But that is not always the case, warns Dr. Varro E. Tyler of Purdue University School of Pharmacy and Pharmacal Sciences. Hemlock is an herb, but it also is a deadly poison. Ask Socrates. Ephedra, also known as ma huang, can cause heart problems. Comfrey, borage, and coltsfoot, all in common use until recently, can cause severe liver problems.

Here are some of Dr. Tyler's guidelines for safe, effective use of herbs.

1. **Let your doctor know what you're doing.**
2. **Consult scientific literature to determine whether an herb is good for a particular condition. Dr. Tyler often credits German studies, reported by the government Commission E, as reliable herbal information, in addition to referring people to his own book, *The Honest Herbal*, 3rd edition.**
3. **When possible, buy products that guarantee standardized potencies on the label. And buy from reputable, reliable companies.**
4. **Read the label carefully. Make sure that the ingredients you want are in the herbal medication and in the dosage you need.**
5. **Buy in stores that sell a lot of product because you want fresh herbs. Many lose their potency as they age—whether in your cabinet or on a store shelf.**
6. **If you experience side effects or unusual reactions like rashes, stop taking the herb immediately.**

says. As an extra added bonus, psyllium can cut cholesterol, too. For regularity, though, you have to use it, um, regularly. Follow the instructions on the label.

Feeling more vital. Studies show that taking ginseng, along with a multivitamin, lifts spirits and, in general, makes a man feel better, Dr. Tyler says. It's a tonic. Of the many products on the market, the concentration of ginsenosides may vary. Buy a standardized extract that contains 4 percent of the active ingredient ginsenosides, and follow the dosage on the label, he says.

An herb called Siberian ginseng, which really is not a member of the true ginseng family, works similarly, says Terry Willard, Ph.D., herbalist and director of the Wild Rose School of Natural Healing in Calgary, Alberta, Canada. Dr. Willard suggests taking from 500 to 1,000 milligrams of Siberian ginseng twice daily.

Thinking faster, feeling harder. Some herbal experts see ginkgo biloba as a male godsend. Not only does it seem to help solve erectile difficulties in some men but also it improves cognition (thinking ability). It does this by increasing blood flow without affecting blood pressure. It is one of the most frequently prescribed drugs in Germany and France, says Adriane Fugh-Berman, M.D., former head of field investigations for the Office of Alternative Medicine at the National Institutes of Health in Bethesda, Maryland, and author of *Alternative Medicine*. It has been shown to help with memory problems, concentration difficulties, depression, and dizziness.

For the best results, take ginkgo in a 50-to-1 extract, says Dr. Willard. That means the label should say that it contains 24 percent flavonoid glycosides—the active ingredient that increases blood flow.

Raising the Root

Man has forever been on a quest for the magical pill, drink, or salve that will induce an impressive erection reliably. And over several thousand years, certain herbs have gained a sexy reputation. So before you try prescription medicine or injecting hormones, you might want to try a few herbal approaches, says botanist and herbalist Dr. James Duke.

Here's Dr. Duke's rundown on a number of plants purported to pump up your penis, as described in his book *The Green Pharmacy*. You wouldn't rub these on it, by the way. You'd consume them—as tea, or in capsules or some other form.

Anise. Contains estrogen-like substances that reportedly increase male libido. Estrogen is a female hormone. Oddly, some female hormones seem to have male hormone effects when taken by men. That may be what's happening with anise.

Ashwaganda. Try this root, an alleged erection-arouser from the traditional folk medicine of India. But it's meant to be taken occasionally, not daily.

Cardamom. This common spice contains a central nervous system stimulant. Does it have any sexual effect? Arab tradition holds that it does. It can't hurt to sprinkle a little into your tea or coffee.

Fava bean. This contains a nice dose of L-dopa, a drug that, when taken in large enough doses, produces pri-

It's best not to exceed 240 milligrams daily, warns botanist and herbalist James Duke, Ph.D., of Washington, D.C., in his book *The Green Pharmacy*. Higher doses can cause diarrhea and irritability.

Shrinking an enlarged prostate. Saw palmetto helps, Dr. Tyler says. However, he warns that we should not self-diagnose prostate

apism—a painful, persistent, unwanted erection. Chances are that you'll never eat enough fava beans to have that problem. But a manly 8- to 16-ounce serving might be a real pick-me-up.

Ginger. Or Mary Ann? One or the other always turned *us* on. Arab folk medicine says that this will make your putter perk up. Some scientists believe that ginger improves sperm's swimming ability.

Wild oats. It works for stallions, and some studies say that human males get friskier, too, when fed wild oats. You'll find the Latin name for wild oats, *avena sativa,* listed as an ingredient on bottles of some very expensive formulations for men in health food stores.

Wolfberry. This has been shown to raise testosterone levels. That's not going to help with erections unless testosterone levels are really low.

Yohimbine. It works for some men some of the time, but the side effects are dangerous—including anxiety, increased heart rate, elevated blood pressure, and hallucinations. If you want the effects of yohimbine, ask your doctor for the prescription version, yohimbine hydrochloride, which contains only the active ingredient and seems to have far fewer side effects than the herb. According to controlled scientific studies, one-third of men taking yohimbine get the desired result.

tains 85 to 95 percent fatty acids and sterols. The fatty acids and sterols contain the plant medicine that benefits prostate tissue, so you want to be sure that you're getting a potent percentage of that. A usual dose is 80 to 160 milligrams twice daily, says Dr. Tyler.

Coping with depression.
Several active principles in the herbal remedy Saint-John's-wort are proving to be effective antidepressants for mild to moderate depression. It doesn't work instantly, though. Although it can be taken as a tea, it is best consumed in capsule or tablet form, standardized on the basis of hypericin, a marker, not necessarily an active component, advises Dr. Tyler. Follow label dosage directions carefully. The antidepressant effect should be evident within six weeks.

Solving stomach upset.
Ginger, the cooking spice and the flavor in real ginger ale, is a great stomach-soother and a pleasant motion-sickness preventive, says Dr. Tyler. This root can stop nausea quickly. You can make a tea with ½ to 1 teaspoon grated fresh ginger, or with 1 teaspoon ground ginger.

Warning: It does have a pepperlike bite. If you prefer, you can eat some crystallized ginger candy. Or drink real ginger ale (not "artificially flavored"). For motion-sickness prevention, take the cure 20 to 25 minutes before you take off, of course.

Sleeping easier.
Valerian is a mild tranquilizer that has been shown to help people fall asleep. And it doesn't leave you with the morning hangover associated with other sleeping pills, Dr. Tyler says. Valerian smells terrible, so it is better taken in capsule form than in a tea. Follow the instructions on the label, advises Dr. Tyler.

problems. Let the doctor do that, then discuss alternative treatments, he advises. If the problem *is* enlarged prostate, then consider the herb. In Germany, doctors prescribe saw palmetto and other herbal remedies nearly 90 percent of the time to relieve enlarged prostates.

Read saw palmetto labels carefully, Dr. Tyler advises, and purchase a brand that con-

Laughter

How to Be a Good Humor Man

Ever since the late *Saturday Review* editor Norman Cousins published *Anatomy of an Illness*, documenting how he used laughter in combination with his therapy to overcome a potentially fatal connective tissue disease, the medical profession has given the therapeutic power of humor a serious second look. One study found that people who watched a 60-minute comedy video boosted production of white blood cells—the ones that fight disease—by 39 percent and decreased levels of a hormone that triggers stress by 46 percent. In another study in 1996, one of the leading researchers in this area found that blood samples from men who viewed a humorous video contained increased levels of a chemical that fights viruses and strengthens the immune system.

But the researcher, Lee Berk, Dr. P.H., clinical preventive care clinician and assistant research professor of pathology and laboratory medicine at Loma Linda University School of Medicine in Loma Linda, California, does not take credit for first recognizing the healthful benefits of good humor. He points to a much earlier document: the Bible. "A merry heart doeth good like a medicine: but a broken spirit drieth the bones," we are told in Proverbs 17:22.

Anatomy of a Mirther

Someone tells a joke. The corners of your mouth curl up. Your face crinkles. Depending on the vintage and virtue of the humor (Henny Youngman, Richard Pryor, Jerry Seinfeld),

you emit a chuckle, giggle, chortle, a heh-heh, or a deep-bellied riotous guffaw. That laughter is the behavioral response to a perceptual process known as humor, explains Patty Wooten, R.N., of Santa Cruz, California, who performs as a professional clown for hospital patients and is the author of *Compassionate Laughter*.

She breaks down the physical action into two stages similar to exercise: the arousal phase, when all physiological hell breaks loose; and the resolution phase, when that guffaw simmers down and you return to a normal resting rate. During vigorous sustained laughter, your heart rate can rise as high as 120 beats per minute. Respiration also jumps, resulting in faster and deeper breaths. And that sends more oxygen into your blood. A variety of muscle groups become active: diaphragm, abdominal, facial—even legs, arms, and back muscles when it's a real knee-slapper. This increases the flow of blood throughout the body. All in all, laughter gives you a good physical workout. In fact, researchers have found that 100 laughs are the aerobic equivalent of 10 minutes on a rowing machine. And, as we all know by now, aerobic exercise is one of the best ways to keep our hearts hardy and assure us years more of laughter.

As for the mind, Wooten says, a good yuk "helps us change our perspective on our problems and enables us to develop an attitude of detachment, a sense of self-protection, and control over our environment and other nasty negative influences."

He Who Laughs Last . . .

All of this might suggest that there are a number of short-term benefits of humor to body, mind, and soul. But are there really long-term effects? This was the question that tickled Richard Haude, Ph.D., professor emeritus of psychology at the University of Akron in Ohio. Based on the short-term pluses, he and his colleagues speculated that "it is possible that a jocular nature and an ongoing appreciation of humor may facilitate successful survival into older adulthood." In other words, they figured a good punch line could add to your life line.

To test their hypothesis, Dr. Haude and his colleagues asked 33 older adults with a mean age of 72.3 to rate themselves and a deceased sibling (mean age at death was 64.6) on a scale that evaluates one's sense of humor. The results showed that the surviving siblings had a better sense of humor than their dead relatives. Though he admits the data are limited, Dr. Haude says the study shows that "if you appreciate humor to a greater extent than somebody else, you're likely to live a little longer."

Now this is all well and good for a person who is a natural-born comedian, but what about the person who cannot make others laugh? Is there hope for the humor-impaired? Michelle Gayle Newman, Ph.D., assistant professor of psychology at Pennsylvania State University in University Park, thinks so. In a study she conducted, she found that two groups of people—one that tended to use humor to cope with stress and another group that didn't—both benefited positively from using humor during exposure to a stressful film. In this study, all participants, even those who didn't have a sense of humor, demonstrated fewer stress reactions to the film when they used humor coping than participants who did not use humor coping. As a result of her study, Dr. Newman now believes that "humor can be learned."

So keep practicing those punch lines.

The Mirthful Medicine Chest

If you wait for something funny to happen to lift your spirits and lengthen your life, you may be frowning a long time. In these serious times, you have to be proactive about soliciting joyfulness, says Dr. Lee Berk of Loma Linda University School of Medicine. "You have to push your behavior," he says. "When you do, your brain chemistry will change and your emotions will follow."

For just such down-in-the-dumps situations, he suggests keeping a well-stocked arsenal of laugh-makers on hand. His humor apothecary would include:

- *A joke book.* Anything by Dave Barry or Rodney Dangerfield. But really, select the humor that humors you.

- *A collection of comedy videos,* such as any of Robin Williams's live performances. But again, it's your call.

- *Funny films.* Once again, the choice is yours. Dark humor like *The War of the Roses* might fit the bill on certain occasions, while *National Lampoon's Animal House* or the Marx Brothers golden oldies could elicit guffaws on others.

- *A little red clown's nose.* For real. Go buy one at a costume shop. Put it on and look in the mirror. If that doesn't crack you up, nothing will. As for wearing it in public, we take no responsibility for the repercussions.

- *Mad* magazine. Is there a man alive who secretly or quite publicly did not go through pre- and postadolescence reading the borders of *Mad* behind his biology textbook? And, now more than ever, we could all learn from Alfred E. Neuman's motto: "What, me worry?"

You may never make it to the open mike night at your local comedy club, but you could still be standing to hear the next generation of stand-up comedians.

Medical Testing

Taking Inventory of Your Health

Ken Goldberg, M.D., often likens himself to a car mechanic who is trying to salvage cars after they've been run into the ground and their engines have burned up. "I see these men who have neglected themselves for years. Now they come to me with tons of damage and want to be repaired," groans the founder and director of the Male Health Institute in Dallas and author of *How Men Can Live As Long As Women.* "Maybe if men had inspection stickers on themselves, they'd take as good care of their own bodies as they do their cars and trucks."

Men should start getting basic medical tests in their twenties, says Dr. Goldberg, and add tests as needed as they get older. The following is a general guideline. Talk to your doctor about tailoring a medical test schedule that specifically fits your medical needs.

The Baseline: Your Twenties

The problem with guys in their twenties, says Dr. Goldberg, is that they're invincible. "Or at least they think they are," he says. While it's true that you're less likely to have serious health problems at this younger stage in life, now is a great time to map out a lifestyle plan to help you prevent diseases in the future. You can also catch any potential problems, such as high blood pressure, in their infancy and stop them there, says Dr. Goldberg.

To head off future health woes, doctors recommend getting the following tests starting when you're in your twenties.

History and physical: See your doctor for a history and physical every three years until you turn 40, suggests Dr. Goldberg. Then switch to every two years until you are 50, when you should start getting them annually. It's here that your physician learns all about you and your family history: health problems dating back to childhood; any current medical conditions such as allergies, diseases, or medications; lifestyle factors, such as whether you drink or smoke; and any other pertinent information.

Blood pressure: Have your blood pressure checked every three years until you turn 40; then switch to every two years, says John Coulehan, M.D., professor of medicine and preventive medicine at the State University of New York at Stony Brook School of Medicine. "This might be one of the most important screenings you can have done," Dr. Coulehan says. "There are absolutely no symptoms to high blood pressure. Untreated, it can lead to heart attack, stroke, kidney failure, and many other problems." To refresh your memory, blood pressure is read in two numbers, the top number being systolic; the bottom, diastolic. Systolic pressure measures the force of blood flow at its peak. Diastolic measures blood pressure at its lowest point. A normal reading is around 120/80 millimeters of mercury (read as "120 over 80"). Consistent readings above 140/90 are high.

Blood count: Have your blood count done every three years, until you reach 40; then have it tested every two years, suggests Dr.

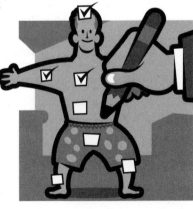

Coulehan. This test measures the quality of your blood and the levels of three types of blood cells needed for optimum health: red cells, which carry oxygen; white cells, which fight infection; and platelets, which help with blood clotting. Low levels of red blood cells can be a sign of anemia, a major cause of fatigue.

Urinalysis: Have a urine test done every three years until you reach 40; then switch to every two years, says Dr. Goldberg. Give your doctor a paper cup with a small urine sample, and he can tell you how well your kidneys function, whether you're drinking enough water, whether you have any kidney stones or prostate or urinary tract infections, and even if you have diabetes or some cancers.

Tuberculosis test: You should have a tuberculin skin test every three to five years throughout your life, Dr. Goldberg suggests. Tuberculosis has gone from the history books to the newspaper headlines. And today's strains are harder to fight with traditional medications, making early detection essential. Men are twice as likely to get tuberculosis as women. You are particularly vulnerable if you live in crowded conditions or work in the teaching or health-care professions.

Cholesterol screening: You should have your cholesterol—or lipid profile—screened every three years until your 40th birthday; then switch to every two years, suggests Dr. Goldberg. Cholesterol screenings will tell you several things: Your level of "bad" low-density lipoprotein (LDL) cholesterol, which is known to form plaque on artery walls; your level of "good" high-density lipoprotein (HDL) cholesterol, which appears to prevent plaque buildup; and the triglycerides in your blood, which are body fats that, when present at high levels, can contribute to heart disease risk. Ideally, you should aim for total cholesterol of no more than 200 milligrams per deciliter and LDL cholesterol of no more than 130 milligrams per deciliter. HDL should be at least 35 milligrams per deciliter, but more is better. Triglyceride levels should register under 200 milligrams per deciliter.

Eye exam: You should have your vision checked every three years until you reach 40 and then every two years thereafter, just to be

The Seven Signs

No matter what your age, it's important to keep an eye out for the seven warning signs of cancer, says Dr. Ken Goldberg of the Male Health Institute. If you notice one of these signs or symptoms, make an appointment with your doctor right away. The sooner you catch cancer, the better your chance for successful treatment. Here they are.

1. **Change in bowel or bladder habits, such as a thinner stool, a change in color of urine or stool, or a change in frequency**
2. **A sore that doesn't heal**
3. **Unusual bleeding or discharge in your ejaculate, in your stool, or in your urine, or if you're coughing up blood**
4. **A lump or thickening anywhere on your body, particularly under your arm or in or around your chest**
5. **Prolonged indigestion or difficulty swallowing**
6. **Obvious change in a wart or mole**
7. **Nagging cough or hoarseness**

sure that you're seeing as clearly as possible, says Dr. Coulehan.

Testicular self-exam: If you're younger than 40, you should check your testicles every month, but it doesn't hurt to keep checking them monthly even after you are 40. "Testicular cancer is the most common solid cancer in men younger than 35," Dr. Goldberg says. (See "Do It Yourself" on page 64 for how to do a testicular self-exam.)

Electrocardiogram: You should get a baseline electrocardiogram done at every decade throughout your life, says Dr. Goldberg. This test uses electrodes on your wrists and ankles and chest to determine the electrical activity of your heart. Any abnormalities will alert your doctor that there may be some form of heart disease in progress and that he should perform further tests.

HIV test: While not recommended as part of routine screening tests, if you feel that you are at risk for HIV because of your sexual practices or intravenous drug use, you should be tested regularly. "But having a clean AIDS test is not a license to act irresponsibly," warns Dr. Coulehan. "A negative test does not mean that you are invulnerable to future infection. Obviously, you will need to practice safe sex."

Your Thirties

If you skipped over the section "The Baseline: Your Twenties," go back immediately and read it. Your health program for your thirties includes those same tests. In certain cases, you may want to add the following test, suggests Dr. Coulehan.

Glaucoma test: If you have a family history of glaucoma, start testing now, says Dr. Coulehan. Otherwise, you can begin testing at 40, and test every two years from there.

Your Forties

Age 40 is when it's time to step up your tests, generally getting them every other year instead of every three. It's also time to start tending to your lower half. Your risk for colon cancer rises sharply when you hit your midforties, and your risk for prostate cancer increases as well. In addition to the other aforementioned tests, get this test now, suggests Dr. Goldberg. He also notes that race and personal or family history of illness can change the timing and frequency of medical tests.

Rectal exam: Nobody wants one. Every 40-plus man needs one every year, says

Do It Yourself

Let's be honest. Even if you like your doctor, nobody really likes going because of the inconvenience, if for no other reason. Thanks to the innovations of modern technology, there are plenty of tests you can—and in some cases should—do in the comfort of your own home. Here are the key ones that experts recommend.

Check your testicles. Simply place your index and middle fingers underneath your testicles and your thumbs on top. Then gently roll your testicles between your fingers. They should feel like shelled, hard-boiled eggs. In addition, each time you get a physical, your doctor should give you an exam.

Inspect your skin. There are 900,000 nonmelanoma skin cancers diagnosed each year in the United States. You should do a quick inventory of your skin for any persistent sores, new molelike growths, or changes in existing moles each month.

Watch your sugar. If you have diabetes, your doctor may suggest that you monitor your blood sugar levels. You can buy a home monitoring system from most drugstores. Otherwise, have your doctor check your blood sugar levels when you have your regular blood work done.

Check your chest and glands. Breast cancer is not

Dr. Goldberg. A digital rectal exam (DRE)—in which your doctor inserts a gloved, lubricated finger into your rectum to feel your prostate—is your best line of defense against prostate cancer.

Your Fifties and Beyond

Not much changes between 40 and 50, so long as you're continuing your regular tests about every two years. At age 50, start getting physicals annually and continue getting the

exclusive to women, warns Dr. Ken Goldberg of the Male Health Institute. "Check the area around your nipples and under your arms for lumps or thickenings monthly. And while you're at it, check the glands in your neck and groin for any tenderness or swelling," he says. If you find any lumps or swelling, have it checked by your doctor.

Test your pressure. This is usually done in the doctor's office. But if you have a history of high blood pressure, it's not a bad idea to have a blood pressure cuff at home, say some doctors. Before using a home device, it's a good idea to take it to your doctor first to make sure that you are using and reading it correctly.

See how you see. Concerned about worsening vision? You can buy an eye chart at most medical supply stores. Hang it on your wall and check your vision from a designated distance.

Check your cholesterol. For $15 to $20 you can buy a finger-stick home cholesterol test from most drugstores.

Screen for HIV. If you are sexually active outside of a long-standing, completely monogamous relationship, consider investing in a home HIV test for your own and your current partner's peace of mind.

look into your rectum and large intestine for polyps, or growths that might signal cancer. The test takes just a few minutes. And don't worry. The sigmoidoscope is so thin and flexible, doctors say that although the test is uncomfortable, it is not painful. If you are at higher risk because of family or personal history, your doctor may recommend more inclusive tests such as colonoscopy or a barium enema at an earlier age.

PSA screening: PSA (prostate-specific antigen) screening is a blood test that checks for a compound that is produced exclusively by the prostate gland. Significant increases in this compound can indicate a problem, such as prostate cancer. You should have this test done every year starting at age 50, says Dr. Goldberg, unless you are at high risk because of your family history or if you are an African-American.

Acing the Test of Life

The final bit of advice doctors give regarding medical tests is don't mistake "good grades" with good health.

"I see people who think that all they need for good health is to pass a battery of medical tests," Dr. Coulehan says. "Absolutely nothing is a substitute for good, healthy living. Without it, all medical tests do is show you how your unhealthy living is taking its toll. People quibble with me whether their cholesterol levels are 220 or 200 while they're smoking a pack of cigarettes a day.

"Live healthfully. Eat less than 30 percent of your calories from fat. Be active," Dr. Coulehan advises. "And have a good relationship with your doctor so that you can put your medical tests, your medical history, and your health habits in perspective."

DREs you started getting in your forties. Just add a couple more tests, and you're set for life, says Dr. Goldberg.

Stool sample: During a DRE, the doctor will also take a tiny sample of stool to test for any traces of blood—a sign of cancer growth or development. Like DREs, this should be done every year, says Dr. Coulehan.

Sigmoidoscopy: Your 50th birthday is a good time to start having this test, and then get it done every five years thereafter, says Dr. Goldberg. A sigmoidoscope is a thin, flexible, lighted instrument that actually lets the doctor

Sex

Doing What's Good for You

Sex is healthy. Admittedly, that's hardly a novel notion. But in an age when you have to find ways to make sex "safe," a little reminder of sex's essentially salutary nature never hurts.

Keep in mind, though, that "healthy" is one thing, "medicinal" is another. True, intercourse does have its direct health benefits. It is, after all, exercise (though it comes in well below golf and sawing wood on the calorie-burning charts). It has an analgesic effect, reducing pain for several hours after the fact, most encouragingly for sufferers of arthritis. And there's evidence that ejaculations on a steady, regular basis make for a healthier prostate.

But sex, as far as anybody knows, doesn't cure cancer. It won't prevent heart disease. We'd love to report that sex will fend off diabetes forever. But that, as a certain jowly ex-president once said, would be wrong.

Still, it's wrong only in its overstatement, not in spirit. Sexual fulfillment *is* a player in the disease-fighting game, not because it cures anything directly but because it's a morale-booster.

Sex is a motivator and a powerful one, according to Aaron Vinik, M.D., Ph.D., director of research at the Diabetes Institute in Norfolk, Virginia. "The contact that sex provides keeps you functioning and involved," Dr. Vinik says. "Sexually inactive people become what I call slothful—apathetic and inactive."

Apathy and inactivity are invitations to disease; they're the antithesis of the disease-free lifestyle. To defy disease, you need to exchange those two losers for a couple of winners: inspiration and action. A lusty sex life is part of that motivational mix.

"A lot of the depression and withdrawal you see in people with illnesses is because of a loss of sexuality," Dr. Vinik says. "Sex is important to feel whole, to have a healthy outlook, to maintain vibrancy."

Bop till You Drop

There are two ways of looking at the picture. First, robust sexuality keeps you in a better position to stay disease-free. Second, avoiding disease—especially cardiovascular disease and diabetes—is the best thing you can do for your long-term sex life. So not only is sex healthy but also health is sexy.

And while abundant sex won't guarantee that you live to be 96, consider this advice from our experts. As you're preparing to live into your nineties as a result of other information you've gleaned from these pages, schedule in enough sex time.

You're going to want it for the same reasons you want it now. It's a way of having special intimacy with your partner, it's an excellent form of relaxation, and it's the best outlet for your horny desires.

"There's no specific decline in libido with age," says Alan Brauer, M.D., founder of the Brauer Total Care Medical Center in Palo Alto, California, and co-author of *ESO: The New Promise of Pleasure for Couples in Love.* "Sexual interest doesn't change, even in men in their eighties and nineties." And even at that age,

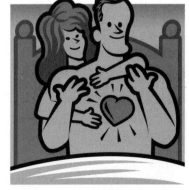

you'll probably be not only willing but also able. "Erection capacity in healthy men should remain—in fact, does remain—into their nineties," Dr. Brauer says.

The key word there is *healthy*. Age per se doesn't wilt your weapon, no matter what you've heard to the contrary. But disease does.

"The graph that shows progressive increases of erectile

dysfunction with advancing age is from data taken from hospital populations, people with vascular disease, heart disease, diabetes, alcoholism, and so forth," Dr. Vinik points out. "You take a population of healthy aging people, and that's not going to occur."

Have Sex Forever

That's not to say that everything about your sex life is going to stay the same as you get older. It never stayed the same your first 50 years, so why should your last 50 be change-free? The problem is that younger men, looking ahead, see change leading only to some kind of feeble approximation of the real thing.

Not so. "Your physical responsiveness is altered to a degree, but not radically," says Dr. Brauer.

So if you want to have sex for the rest of your life, don't focus on your physical changes. Focus on the things you can do to make sure that you keep having sex for the rest of your life.

Do it or eschew it. The secret to healthy sex in your sixties or seventies and beyond is to have healthy sex in your fifties and forties and before. "It's very difficult for a man who pretty much stopped having sex in his fifties to start it up again when he's 75," Dr. Brauer says.

That's because sex is plumbing. The more the blood flows to the penis, the more it wants to. "If you stop having sexual relationships, the disuse leads to atrophy of the blood vessels in the penis and impairment of blood flow to the penis," Dr. Vinik says. Translation: Your equipment shuts down, taking your sex life along with it.

Go solo. Those times in your life when you might be partnerless are no reason to let

Why Love Feels So Good

The buxom brunette brushes against you, and immediately you know that the chemistry is right. That's not just a saying. There _is_ chemistry involved, says Theresa Crenshaw, M.D., a sex therapist in San Diego and the author of _The Alchemy of Love and Lust_ and other books.

How we relate to others—and just the act of relating—causes changes in our body chemistry, which, in turn, influences our health and well-being. Love and sex (every man's favorite subjects) offer a great example.

Phenylethylamine, a naturally occurring hormone, gives you a natural high and is an antidepressant besides, Dr. Crenshaw says. Its levels rise and fall with feelings of love and reach crescendo upon orgasm.

Other "love drugs" help keep us together once we pass beyond infatuation, Dr. Crenshaw says. Among those are the hormones oxytocin, prolactin, and vasopressin. Oxytocin is the major bonding hormone. Levels shoot sky-high in women when they orgasm. They want to cuddle then. Levels rise less dramatically in men in response to intimate and affectionate touch. And then, when we are separated from our lover, we are likely to experience some withdrawal symptoms and cravings, Dr. Crenshaw says. Ah, the stuff of love.

the plumbing back up. "I recommend that men maintain a certain frequency of erection and orgasm," Dr. Brauer says. "At least two orgasms a week have been found to be associated with improved physical health and longevity. And that can be achieved with solo sex if that's what it takes."

You won't be the only guy using masturbation to keep his equipment in working order.

"Two-thirds of married men are doing some kind of regular self-stimulation," Dr. Brauer says. "That can and probably should continue throughout life."

Ask for a helping hand. At 20, your erection may happen from just thinking about her disrobing. At 35, it may happen by watching her disrobe. At 60, it happens if she fondles your genitals, robed or not. "Direct stimulation is very important for a man in his middle or later years," Dr. Brauer says. "And not only direct stimulation but continuous stimulation."

That shouldn't be a problem since you don't often hear men grumbling, "What a drag. I have to put up with a lot of stroking and licking from her before the real action." But Dr. Brauer suggests that you find tactful ways to instruct her on this since she may misinterpret the new requirement as an insult to her sex appeal.

Stay high and dry. Fact: You'll deliver less ejaculate as you get older. And sometimes you won't ejaculate at all, a change that's considerately accompanied by less urge to do so. "Enjoy the process without feeling that you necessarily have to ejaculate to finish it off," Dr. Brauer says. Having orgasms without ejaculating may allow you to have this sort of climax more frequently than if you did ejaculate, he adds.

Check your hormones. Your hormone levels don't generally drop enough with age to cramp your sexual style. But sometimes they do, and you may feel the need to talk to your doctor about getting testosterone supplements, often in the form of a skin patch you apply to your body.

"If your testosterone levels are lower than average for your age, you may benefit from supplementation," Dr. Brauer says. "In fact, some doctors believe that if your testosterone levels are lower than average and you are in your midthirties, supplements may be desirable. It may also be worthwhile to make sure

---

The Last Gasp

If your penis starts developing limp habits, there is some reason to be concerned. Blood that's not flowing well to your penis may not be flowing well elsewhere. And ignoring that fact could be fatal, says Dr. Aaron Vinik of the Diabetes Institute.

"The penis is a divining rod," Dr. Vinik says. "It's very sensitive. Impotence is an important warning of other complications." So pay attention to ongoing incidents of impotence, and don't hesitate to check with your doctor. It's a warning signal, Dr. Vinik says.

---

that other hormones are also at a reasonable level. Other hormones to check are thyroid and adrenal since these, too, can have an influence on sexual interest and response."

Call a mechanic. If technical difficulties beyond your control do keep you from getting erections in your later years, take advantage of some tools available for men with erection problems. The ideas of using a vacuum pump to draw blood into the penis, or injecting an erection-producing substance directly into the penis before sex, might have seemed weird a few decades ago but are now increasingly common among diabetics and others. A new device known as Muse inserts a rice grain–size soft pellet of the erection-enhancing substance called alprostadil one inch up the urethra. "It is helpful for some men with unstable natural erections," says Dr. Brauer.

"For a certain number of men with erection insecurity, a mechanical device is wonderful," Dr. Brauer says.

And in case you're wondering, the shots are relatively simple. "During genital examinations, we give the patient a little pinch," says Dr. Vinik. "When he asks what that was all about, we tell him that's all he'll feel when he gives himself the shot. It's a piece of cake."

Sleep

Never a Waste of Time

You don't hear a lot of guys these days bragging about how much they sleep. Your typical male looks at sleep and sees an unproductive waste of time, an indulgence of the newborn, the retired, and the slothful.

Sleep experts, on the other hand, see it as a restorative daily health tonic, an ally of the alert, the ambitious, and the long-lived.

In fact, researchers suspect and are investigating a direct link between sleep deprivation and disease. There's already at least one study supporting the widespread suspicion among sleep specialists that people who don't sleep very long don't live very long. Several researchers have connected insufficient sleep with less-efficient immune system functioning, possibly via a reduction in the activity of NK cells—the "natural killers" that go after invading viruses.

Disorders and Disdain

A serious sleep disorder such as sleep apnea can quadruple the risk of heart attacks and triple the risk of stroke, even in otherwise healthy men.

But the troublemaking tendencies of inadequate sleep more often come down to basic military strategy. In your war on disease, like any other war, rested troops fight best.

Take stress, for example. While it's still not proved that inadequate sleep causes stress, it certainly sabotages your ability to handle your daily dose of it. "If you're poorly rested,

you're likely to find stressful situations to be even more so. And the relationship between stress and health is fairly clear," says sleep researcher Michael Vitiello, Ph.D., professor in the department of psychiatry and behavioral sciences at the University of Washington School of Medicine in Seattle.

Stress isn't the only one of life's little challenges your sleep-swindled brain has a problem with. Your reaction skills also take a hit when you cheat your sleep.

"Relatively small amounts of sleep deprivation will quickly affect your alertness and psychomotor performance," says Michael Bonnet, Ph.D., professor of neurology at Wright State University School of Medicine in Dayton, Ohio, and director of the Sleep Laboratory at the Dayton Veterans Affairs Medical Center. "You become less responsive, especially in a sedentary situation, such as driving."

Small wonder, then, that sleepiness is second only to drunkenness as a cause of fatal single-car accidents. All things considered, getting yourself killed in a car crash is not a recommended strategy for avoiding disease.

So why do so many guys shirk their sleep duties? Some suffer from one of the more than 80 disorders dogging our sleep. The most well-known is insomnia—difficulty in getting to sleep or staying there—which haunts women more than men. The most serious, though, is sleep apnea. And it can be a killer. Its top targets are men between ages 30 and 60, especially if they're overweight. One study found that 24 percent of healthy middle-age men had sleep apnea.

With sleep apnea, you literally (and repeatedly) stop breathing when you are asleep. It's actually your body's rescue plan to keep arousing you so that you can breathe again. But the constant waking, even though it's so brief that you won't even remember, deprives you of the sleep you need. Your sleeping hours are virtually worthless; hence, your waking life is virtually nonfunctional. "And that's life-threatening," says Michael Stevenson, Ph.D., a psychologist and sleep specialist at the North Valley Sleep Disorders Center in Mission Hills, California. "It can get bad enough to increase your blood pressure and your risk for stroke and heart attack, not to mention automobile accidents and injuries on the job."

So if you snore (harmless in itself, but also a possible clue to apnea) and you find yourself constantly waking up sleepy and staying that way all day, pay attention. See a sleep specialist, says Dr. Stevenson. Sleep apnea is treatable.

Serious as apnea can be, the most common reason that men don't sleep enough is . . . well, that they just don't sleep enough. Ask almost any man and he'll tell you that he functions just fine on limited Zzzs, thank you. But there's a difference between functioning well and just functioning, according to Dr. Vitiello. "I'd never argue with someone who says he can get by on four or five hours sleep," he says. "But his very choice of words condemns him. He's *getting by*."

The A to Z of Zzzs

Sound sleep, then, is an essential element of your overall health strategy. But let's face it, putting long life ahead of live Leno may take some adjusting. As Dr. Stevenson puts it, "You have to work at sleeping well." Here's how.

Get steady. Your "circadian rhythm" is simply the pattern of biological functions (such as the release of certain hormones or changes in body temperature and metabolic rate) that vary with how and when you feel sleepy or alert. The first commandment of circadian rhythm obedience is to keep regular sleeping hours, say sleep researchers. You sleep best when you go to bed at about the same time every night and wake up about the same time every morning.

Haphazard sleeping schedules, on the other hand, can sabotage your circadian rhythm. "Your body temperature does not go up and down as much if you keep a random sleep schedule," Dr. Bonnet says. "So you get into this zombie state where you never feel very alert or very sleepy either."

Stay steady. Why do we sleep late on weekends? Because we can.

Bad idea, Dr. Stevenson says. "The part of your brain that generates sleep doesn't know the difference between Wednesday and Saturday," he points out. "When you sleep in on Saturday and Sunday, you push your sleep cycle forward. It's better to sleep consistently seven days a week."

Catch up on the front end. It'll happen. An important deadline—or a more important party—is going to cut into your sleep time. You can make up for some of that lost sleep (but never all of it) the next night. But do it by going to bed earlier, rather than waking up much later than usual, says Dr. Stevenson. Otherwise, you're sleeping right through your circadian rhythm's wake-up call. And then all you're catching up on is lousy, unrestorative sleep. Besides, Dr. Stevenson says, "what matters is how you sleep over the long haul. What you do in a single night is less important."

Ease your way down. You don't bounce your two-year-old on your knee all evening, then throw him straight into the crib and expect him to sleep. He needs to relax first. So do you, if you want healthy sleep. "Give yourself a half-hour or 60 minutes to fade out," Dr. Stevenson says. "You're entering another part of your life, and you can't do it in an instant. You need to withdraw slowly."

You know best what you find relaxing. By definition, it can't be something potentially upsetting. No checkbook-balancing. No doing your income taxes. Television works for some but upsets others. Remember that a lot of tried-and-true sleep-inducers—such as a warm bath or a glass of milk—probably work because you find them relaxing.

Count sheep. We're serious. Dr. Stevenson suggests a sleep-baiting technique you can do once your head hits the pillow. "Keep your eyes open, focus on deep breathing, and try to stay awake rather than try to go to sleep," he says. "Then visualize something you find calming—like fishing on a lake." Or counting sheep? You bet. "That old cliché is actually distracting, relaxing, and kind of hypnotic," Dr. Stevenson says.

Wait until you're sleepy. So you're not sleepy, you say? That's fine, but stay out of the bedroom until you are. That's especially true when you want to sleep but can't. "You start to see your bedroom as this place of torture where you can't sleep," Dr. Stevenson says. "If you're not sleepy, you should get out of there."

In fact, sleep experts urge you to use your bedroom for nothing but sleeping—no television, no writing desk, no rowing machine. Of course, they make an exception for sexual relations, but only if the sexual relationship is going well. Hmmm . . .

Keep naps short. There's actually a downward blip in your alertness level around midafternoon, a fine time for a restorative power nap. But keep it limited to a half-hour to an hour, says Timothy Roehrs, Ph.D., director of research at the Henry Ford Hospital Sleep Disorders and Research Center in Detroit. Longer naps can actually work against your circadian rhythm.

And any time spent napping is time you won't sleep at night. "A nap is a perfectly good thing if you can deal with that trade-off," Dr. Vitiello says.

How Much Is Enough?

Different guys need different amounts of sleep. So how do you know how much is right for you? Sorry, there's no standard formula. But there are tests you can take to find out. And don't worry: They're strictly pass-fail.

The feelings test: Drowsiness during the day or early evening is a dead giveaway that you need more sleep. The problem is that you may never slow down long enough to find it out. So schedule some quiet time and pay attention. "If you fall asleep reading or just sitting quietly before your usual bedtime, you're not getting enough sleep," says Dr. Michael Stevenson of the North Valley Sleep Disorders Center.

The alarm clock test: Did you use your alarm clock this morning? "Anybody who answers yes to that question is at least partially sleep-deprived," says Dr. Michael Bonnet of Wright State University School of Medicine. The idea is that if you're allowing yourself the right amount of sleep, you should wake up just before the alarm goes off.

"Start going to bed a half-hour earlier this week, and if your alarm is still waking you up, keep going to bed a half-hour earlier each week until you find the point where you don't need an alarm," Dr. Bonnet recommends.

The max-out test: Next vacation, do some sleep research on yourself. A common study technique is to put volunteers in bed for 10 or more hours a night for weeks at a time to see how long they'll sleep when they have more time than they need to do it. Try it. When you wake up, see how long you slept. That's how much sleep you need, says Dr. Timothy Roehrs of the Henry Ford Hospital Sleep Disorders and Research Center. If you're like most study subjects, it'll be around 8 hours.

Spirituality

Dr. God's Prescription

Want to live forever? Get religion.

The world's major religions promise eternal life. They don't all agree, though, on exactly how we get from here to eternity. But in a nice little cosmic twist, it turns out that spiritual beliefs may well delay our journey to the unknown, allowing us to shuffle along on this mortal coil longer. Numerous studies have suggested that aspects of spirituality contribute to better health, better quality of life, and yes, even longer years.

Just what is this spirituality thing? It is not the same as religiosity. True, religious people are spiritual, but spiritual people are not all religious, notes Krista Kurth, Ph.D., a management consultant in Potomac, Maryland, who specializes in spirituality in the workplace.

Dr. Kurth's preferred definition of *spirituality* is "the Divine influence working in the human heart." That's "Divine" with a capital D. For those uncomfortable with the concept of "the Divine," she offers this definition: "the sense that there is something more than us out there that connects us all." Spirituality, she says, is "our recognition of our connection with the Divine," or with that something greater, be it greater consciousness or greater sense of being.

Let's say that you cultivate a sense of connectedness with the Divine. What is it going to do for you? Scientists who've tried to isolate God in the laboratory do have some answers.

Science Weighs In

Religiously active members of the Church of Jesus Christ of Latter-Day Saints (also known as the Mormons) live longer and have half the death rate from heart disease, cancer, and other debilitating diseases compared to the general population, says James Enstrom, Ph.D., associate research professor in the School of Public Health at the University of California, Los Angeles. Dr. Enstrom knows. He has tracked 10,000 active Mormons for 14 years in order to relate their mortality patterns to their lifestyle. Active Mormons do not smoke, do not drink, and attend church regularly. Sure, abstaining from alcohol and tobacco helps. But it's not the whole story.

Church attendance also appears to be a positive health factor. Dr. Enstrom is not sure how church attendance works its magic. However, he says, Mormon or not, people who attend church regularly generally are healthier than those who do not attend church. Dr. Enstrom is pretty sure because he also followed a large general population sample of nonsmoking people (in an effort to replicate the Mormon lifestyle in a non-Mormon population). What happened? "The nonsmoker who attended church regularly was healthier than the nonsmoker who didn't attend church regularly," he says. Research by other investigators has supported these findings.

But what of the spiritual folks who don't attend church? Do they enjoy better health and a better sense of well-being?

Yes, according to the latest research. The "relaxation response" linked with meditation—a practice with multifarious spiritual origins—provides a plethora of health benefits, says Herbert Benson, M.D., associate professor of medicine at Harvard Medical School and the Beth Israel Deaconess Hospital in Boston and author of *Timeless Healing*. Spirituality also advocates a healthier lifestyle and increases social support,

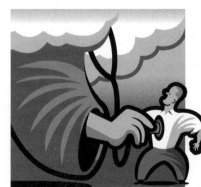

which helps you deal with stress and improves your coping skills.

Positive Energy

In a moment we'll suggest some ways to "inform our lives with spirituality," as Dr. Kurth puts it. But first, what are the other benefits of integrating spirituality into our daily lives or increasing its presence and effect? People whom Dr. Kurth has studied report:

- A sense of deeper meaning, purpose, and direction in life.
- A sense of fulfillment. Maintaining a sense of connectedness and direction is hard work but worth it, says Dr. Kurth, because the process of doing it brings a sense of peace and fulfillment.
- Renewed energy. "People are so burned out in their work lives and in their lives in general," says Dr. Kurth. "Somehow when one taps into that sense of connecting with the Divine, there is a renewed sense of energy."
- Increased feeling of well-being. Psychologists Anne Colby, Ph.D., director of the Henry A. Murray Research Center at Radcliffe College in Cambridge, Massachusetts, and her husband, William Damon, Ph.D., professor of education and director of the Center on Adolescence at Stanford University, conducted a study of people involved in "spiritual work."

These were "people who are highly morally committed, people who are devoting their lives to something they really, deeply believe in," explains Dr. Colby. "Helping the

What Is Spirituality?

Spirituality deals with the big questions. But what exactly is spirituality? That's one of the biggest questions of all.

A review of 250 articles and studies dealing with spirituality revealed that 75 percent defined *spirituality* as a personal philosophy of meaning, say the creators of a course in health-care spirituality at the University of Tennessee, Knoxville, College of Nursing. But this is only part of the story, reported the course creators.

How does one know if he is being spiritual? Management consultant Dr. Krista Kurth says that spiritually inspired actions share the following six traits.

1. They are motivated by an internal attitude of love.

2. They involve giving—or serving others—with no expectation of personal gain. Simple, wholehearted service for others' sake.

3. The elements of compassion and humility are present.

4. The effort involves some degree of difficulty to make because it requires that we transcend our own narrow self-interest.

5. A conscious, ongoing process of growth and learning must take place in order for us to live more fully and express the spiritual aspects.

6. The actions involve spiritual practices or other consciously performed rituals that require commitment, discipline, and effort.

poverty-stricken, fighting for civil rights, things like that."

Dr. Colby and Dr. Damon found that those who do such work for a long period of time tend to be deeply spiritual and have a very optimistic, resourceful, positive approach to life.

They also found that sometimes people can begin working for others for narrow reasons—perhaps pursuing career or business goals—and end up transforming their outlook. They may end up adopting a broader set of moral goals and a more selfless spiritual perspective simply from the process of doing the work and engaging other people as they do it.

What about the benefits of meditation we mentioned earlier?

We know that many American males associate meditation with short, fat, bearded men who wear orange robes. But it needn't be that. Meditation can be cool.

As the body and mind relax in meditation, the brain begins pumping calming chemicals and sending soothing signals that cause our bodies to relax even more. These signals also stave off or even repair the ravages of stress, a known life-threatener and life-shortener, says Dr. Larry J. Feldman of the Pain and Stress Rehabilitation Center. Our blood is less likely to get clumpy and sticky and less likely to gum up artery walls. That translates into heart health. More than that, studies have shown that in the long term, people who regularly practice meditation or some other effective relaxation process develop a much greater tolerance to all sorts of stressors, says Dr. Feldman.

Catching the Spirit

Of course, there's a catch. In this case, two manly traits interfere with spiritual development. First, we are raised to ignore and discount intuition—our inner voice. Second, we are taught to suppress our emotions. On both counts we need to do some unlearning, says Dr. Kurth. Here's how.

Pause and listen. Don't listen only to your reasoning mind. Listen to your inner urges,

Are You a Spiritual Guy?

Management consultant Dr. Krista Kurth teaches that we have opportunities to grow spiritually on four levels: by focusing on the Divine (inviting more spiritual awareness into our lives), on ourselves (living with integrity), on others (building caring relationships), and on creating communities at work.

Rate yourself (– Weak, 0 Average, + Strong) on each of the practices below. You might wish to devote more attention to those on which you rate yourself as weak.

Do you focus on the Divine by:

1. *Engaging in spiritual practices at work, by yourself or with others?*   –   0   +
2. *Recognizing and focusing on the Divine in others? Focusing on the connectedness of life?*   –   0   +
3. *Talking about spiritual values and issues with others? Encouraging openness to the "movement of Spirit"?*   –   0   +
4. *Choosing work in accordance with your values?*   –   0   +

Do you live with integrity by:

5. *Maintaining a positive and accepting attitude toward life and others? Seeing situations as opportunities to learn?*   –   0   +
6. *Engaging in personal reflection and self-improvement?*   –   0   +
7. *Acting with integrity; behaving ethically?*   –   0   +
8. *Maintaining awareness and vigilance over your actions and emotions?*   –   0   +

nudges, leanings, voices. And give yourself permission to act on them, says Dr. Kurth.

Also, make time to just put the world on "pause," Dr. Kurth says. "We get very caught up

Do you build caring relationships by:

9. *Supporting others' growth by encouraging them to explore and live their personal visions?–*   **0**   **+**

10. *Accepting others, having empathy for them, and treating them with love and respect?* **–**   **0**   **+**

11. *Being present, listening receptively, responding to the needs of others and to the situation at hand?*   **–**   **0**   **+**

12. *Speaking and encouraging the truth by communicating openly and honestly with others, and confronting others in a caring, nondenigrating way?*   **–**   **0**   **+**

13. *Supporting others' creativity?*   **–**   **0**   **+**

Do you create communities at work by:

14. *Giving structure to groups and developing policies based on spiritual values?*   **–**   **0**   **+**

15. *Building shared visions and encouraging participation and collaboration at work?*   **–**   **0**   **+**

16. *Creating an organizational culture that embraces diversity, allows for others' self-expression, and encourages open communication?*   **–**   **0**   **+**

17. *Establishing a sense of community and belonging through celebrations, rituals, and fun events?*   **–**   **0**   **+**

18. *Supporting and serving the broader community by providing for organizational participation in community needs?*   **–**   **0**   **+**

19. *Protecting the natural environment by being environmentally conscious and using resources well?*   **–**   **0**   **+**

Note: Dr. Kurth does not recommend imposing your spiritual beliefs on anyone at work. Any discussion of spirituality must be voluntary.

Get emotional. "Listen to your emotions and let your emotions and passions inform what you do," Dr. Kurth says. One definition of *enthusiasm* is "being infused with the spirit of God," she says. Often when we are impassioned, we are connecting with our spiritual essence, she says.

Meditate. Okay, break out those orange robes. Nahhh, we're kidding. The simplest, most basic meditation, says Dr. Kurth, is simply to pause for five minutes and focus attention on nothing but your breathing. Breathe comfortably, deeply, naturally. Don't force it. Just relax and watch your breathing for a few moments. (For more breathing lessons, see Breathing Techniques on page 44.)

Meet Mother Nature. Take quiet walks in natural settings outdoors, says Dr. Kurth. The beauty, vastness, complexity, and seeming omnipresence of nature can be both awe-inspiring and relaxing.

Pray tell. Talking over problems in prayer, turning them over to a higher power, taking decisions into prayerful consideration, is obviously an effort to connect with the Divine. Throughout history many people have found this a helpful spiritual practice, says Dr. Kurth. You might, too.

Make beautiful music. Singing, playing, or listening to inspirational music opens doors to greater spiritual realization, says Dr. Kurth.

Be creative. Working in any of the creative arts can help one discover and develop his spiritual nature. The key here is work that involves inspiration. *Spirit*, says Dr. Kurth, comes from the Latin word meaning "breath," as in "the breath of life." And the word *inspire* comes from the words "in spirit."

with all the events of our lives. And in order to have an intimate connection with some transcendent reality, we have to take time to stop and listen."

Yoga

You Don't Have to Be a Pretzel Man

Yoga claims to be a science—a spiritual science at that.

Interestingly, science has proved many of the medical claims made by yoga to be valid.

Surprised? Most American men are. But then, the only yogis most of us ever knew were Yogi Bear and Yogi Berra. And since the end of the 1960s, it's been easy to dismiss the concept of yoga as some navel-gazing, hippie-dippie waste of time. Not anymore.

Yoga has been shown to be effective in helping treat heart disease, diabetes, back pain, chronic pain, asthma, colitis, arthritis, depressed immune systems, all manner of stress-related illnesses, and more, says Dr. Arthur Brownstein of the University of Hawaii John A. Burns School of Medicine.

Yoga itself is a complex, several-thousand-year-old, multifaceted system of living drawn and adapted from Hindu teachings. Hatha yoga is the style taught most commonly in the West at health clubs and colleges. This consists primarily of focusing attention on the breath and gentle stretches, says Barbara Lang of the Duke University Center for Living.

Saying No to Stress

The greatest and most quickly realized medical benefits seem to derive from the profound calming effect that yoga produces in the mind and body, Dr. Brownstein says. This breaks the debilitating stress cycle, he says. It does this in four ways.

- Through properly and positively aligning body posture through specific positions (known as poses) and placing mental focus on the efforts
- Through slowing, relaxing, and deepening breathing
- Through directing attention inward, peacefully, meditatively
- Through stretching and limbering muscles gently and increasing circulation

A typical hatha yoga class is programmed to take each participant's body through a full range of motion, stretching and strengthening each joint according to its capacity. Regular practice has been shown to ease pain for arthritis sufferers, says Dr. Brownstein. It does this by increasing flexibility—a benefit every practitioner enjoys, and one that makes us feel better.

Saying Yes to Yoga

We can't take you on a full, hour-long yoga session in two short pages, but we'll give you a sampler of a couple of useful exercises and techniques Lang recommends for loosening and limbering your spine, a practice yogis traditionally claim is key to a long life. If you like the gentle stretching and calm inward focus you should experience with these two exercises, consider looking for a class locally. If you have any serious health problems, you will need medical supervision and a yoga instructor who knows how to work with your condition. We can't guarantee that these exercises will bring you a long life, but we do promise they will not hurt, will not turn you into a contortionist, and will not make you look like Plastic Man.

Just as you wouldn't plunge straight into strenuous exercise at the gym without first warming up, you need to prepare for your yoga exercises. Here's how.

See your breath. First, just lie on your back, relax in a comfortable position, and focus on your breathing, says Dr. Larry J. Feldman of the Pain and Stress Rehabilitation Center. Experience it getting slower and deeper. Envision it moving in and out. This is a simple meditation. Do this for a few minutes.

Relaxing meditation is perhaps the most important element of yoga for beginners, says Dr. Brownstein, because most westerners don't know how to relax. "I tell people, if you do nothing but lie there and breathe and relax during the whole class, you will get something out of it. It will be a beneficial experience," he says. The basic deep breathing technique taught in Breathing Techniques (page 44) will help you cultivate a healthy breath. To add the yoga meditation element to it, simply observe the breath moving in and out of your body. "Let your awareness follow the breath," Dr. Brownstein says.

Envision life-sustaining oxygen entering the body and moving into every cell and tissue as you breathe in, Dr. Brownstein says. Feel your muscles relax and tension leave your body as you breathe out, he says.

Equip yourself. To fully concentrate on the exercises, it will help to have a couple of useful items. One is a tape recorder. It helps to record the breathing instructions on a cassette while reading them at a slow pace. Then you can play the tape when you wish to practice the exercises. Second, you'll need some small terry bath towels. Roll a towel and place it beneath your neck as you lie flat on your back—just so it supports the natural curve. Stack folded towels under your head, one at a time, until you find the most comfortable position, the one in which your neck is completely relaxed and not at all strained. You may also wish to place a rolled towel beneath the small of your back for gentle support. Use these in all poses in which lying on your back is necessary, says Dr. Brownstein.

Stop before pain starts. A caution: Never go beyond the edge of "comfortable discomfort," Dr. Brownstein says. Never move into pain. Go to the edge of the pain, right to the place where, if you stretch further, it would begin to hurt, he advises. Imagine yourself breathing into that edge, he says.

Be sure to breathe as you stretch. Don't hold your breath as people do when they experience pain. And don't push yourself into the pain. Don't hurt yourself, says Dr. Brownstein. That defeats the whole purpose because you can tear muscle fibers. And if you do feel it's too hard at any time, simply lie on your back and relax and focus on your breathing. And how hard is that?

Now that you're equipped for a safe and productive yoga session, try these two back limber-ers, says Dr. Brownstein:

Pelvic tilt: Lie on your back, knees bent, feet flat on the floor, arms resting at your sides comfortably. Take a nice, deep breath in, expanding the chest and belly, and exhale. Gently raise your hips off the floor as high as you can without forcing or straining. Your shoulders, upper back, and back of the head should be pressing into the floor. Hold this position for 10 to 20 seconds or as long as you are comfortable, allowing the breath to flow in and out of your body on its own. Then, releasing the position as you breathe out slowly, lower your hips back down to the floor and relax.

You should work toward repeating this movement up to 10 times.

Spinal twist: Lie on your back. Put your arms out perpendicular to your body, palms up. Bend both knees and bring them toward your chest together. Inhale slowly. As you exhale, lower both knees slowly to the floor on one side of your body. Keep your back flat and arms out. Breathe gently and rest in that position for 30 seconds to a minute. Then inhale, and on the exhalation, slowly bring your knees back to the starting position and repeat the movement on the other side of your body. Do three sets at first. Work up to five.

Vitamins

Just Enough of a Good Thing

Vitamins may be the most convoluted health story of the century. First we discover that without them, we die, slowly and painfully from deficiency diseases like scurvy and beriberi. Then we figure that, if a little is good, more is even better. And folks go haywire, popping more pills than Jimi Hendrix on a bad day. Before long we find out that you really can get too much of a good thing, as people succumb to the side effects of vitamin overdose—like liver damage from too much vitamin D. And now, nearly 100 years after we first heard about vitamins, we're still searching for middle ground.

We know for certain that in the proper amounts vitamins and their sidekick minerals can dramatically improve our health. What we're finally realizing is that vitamins and minerals alone are not the sole makings for good nutrition. We also need substances known as phytochemicals, such as the flavonoids in red wine that fight heart disease and the carotenoids like lycopene in tomatoes that fight prostate cancer. We need fiber, which keeps us regular, lowers cholesterol, and cuts our risk for colorectal cancer. And we likely need countless other compounds that scientists don't even know about yet. The only way to get all that is from food.

The question then is, Should we take supplements at all? The answer is yes, according to Katherine Tucker, Ph.D., associate professor of nutrition at Tufts University in Boston. For two reasons: First, we're imperfect. Try though we may, most

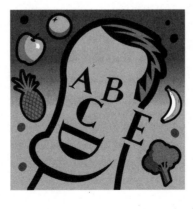

of us still don't eat well enough to get the Daily Values of all the nutrients we need all of the time, especially as we get older, says Dr. Tucker. Second, there are a few nutrients that can provide us extra protection from conditions like heart disease if we take them in doses higher than what we can get from food. Today, most respected nutritionists and experts in the field recommend loading up on fruits and vegetables and taking a multivitamin/mineral supplement to pick up any slack. Obviously, for the best protection, you should take a multi that has enough of the nutrients you need. Here's what to look for.

E-normous Benefits

If you supplement nothing else, supplement vitamin E, advises Dr. Tucker. You've heard by now that vitamin E is an antioxidant. But you likely have no idea just how good this free-radical-fighting nutrient really is. Even researchers have just begun to scratch the surface.

For a quick review, free radicals are simply oxygen molecules just like the ones you're breathing in right now, only they've been damaged—meaning that they lost an electron—by sunlight, pollution, or even your own metabolism. To repair themselves, they steal electrons from your body's healthy molecules, which not only damages your cells but also creates more free radicals. Antioxidants stop this molecular chain of destruction by stepping in and offering their own electrons instead.

Antioxidant action may be most helpful inside your arteries. Scientists have found that it's free-radical damage to your unhealthy low-density lipoprotein cholesterol that makes the stuff stick to your artery walls and eventually clogs them up. Vitamin E is so effective in the fight against hardening of the arteries that when British researchers gave more than 2,000 people with partially blocked coronary arteries either 400 or 800 international units (IU) of vitamin E a day for 18 months, these coronary candidates (of either dose) lowered their risk for nonfatal heart attack by 75 percent.

"The benefits of vitamin E against heart disease are pretty well established," says Dr. Ichiro Kawachi of the Harvard School of Public Health. The Daily Value for vitamin E is only 30 IU, a standard that leading health experts consider far below what you need for disease protection. The problem is that it's practically impossible to get higher, protective amounts of vitamin E from food alone since it's mostly found in fatty oils. You certainly don't want to drink the eight cups of corn oil that it would take to get 400 IU, so Dr. Kawachi recommends taking a supplement of 200 to 400 IU a day instead.

As a bonus, it may make you better in bed. Vitamin E prevents testosterone from breaking down, which keeps your libido up. And it may keep your memory sharp to boot. Though researchers have used only astronomical doses so far (a lot more than anyone should take without a doctor's supervision), vitamin E was able to delay the progression of severe dementia in a group of 341 people with moderately severe Alzheimer's disease, according to a study from Rush Alzheimer's Disease Center in Chicago.

Linus's Legacy

Though the Daily Value for vitamin C is only 60 milligrams, esteemed researcher Linus

---

Easy-to-Swallow Insurance

The best way to fight cancer, heart disease, and countless other conditions is to eat a diet that's low in meat and high in fruits and vegetables, says Dr. Ichiro Kawachi of the Harvard School of Public Health. But for those days that a taco shell is the closest you come to corn, take a multivitamin with 100 percent of the Daily Value for most nutrients or, better yet, supplements targeted for the following amounts of these specific vitamins and minerals, says Dr. Kawachi.

Nutrient	Recommended Amount
Vitamin E	400 international units
Vitamin C	200 to 500 milligrams
Folic acid	400 micrograms (the Daily Value)
Vitamin B$_6$	2 milligrams (the Daily Value)
Vitamin B$_{12}$	6 micrograms (the Daily Value)
Calcium	200 milligrams (provided you're getting about 800 milligrams from three to four servings of low-fat dairy foods a day)
Magnesium	100 to 400 milligrams; people with heart and kidney problems should not take supplemental magnesium
Zinc	15 milligrams (the Daily Value)

Pauling took thousands of milligrams of this powerful antioxidant every day, convinced it would fend off everything from the common cold to cancer. Though Pauling himself lived to be 93, clinical evidence is still inconclusive about what vitamin C can and can't do.

"We have found that high levels of vitamin C seem to protect against cataracts as well," says epidemiologist Paul F. Jacques, D.Sc., associate professor of nutrition at Tufts University. "But we still need more research to understand what levels are beneficial for most people. So far, it looks like more than two times the Daily Value."

Until we know more, a study at the National Institutes of Health indicates that we need 200 to 500 milligrams of vitamin C a day to keep our systems vitamin C–saturated (we lose vitamin C when we urinate). But since it's easy to get vitamin C from food, experts recommend looking for a supplement with about 200 milligrams.

Folic Acid Frenzy

A once-overlooked B vitamin, folic acid has been shoving its way into the spotlight during the past several years—first as a protective agent against life-threatening birth defects of the brain and spine, then as a potential defender against heart attack and stroke.

The U.S. Public Health Service recommends getting the Daily Value of 400 micrograms of folic acid every day, which can be tough unless you eat a lot of greens, drink fortified orange juice, or eat fortified foods. "Food manufacturers are soon going to be fortifying flour and flour products with folic acid much in the way they add thiamin, niacin, and riboflavin today, which should lead to improvements in heart disease rates," Dr. Tucker says. But until you see folic acid appear on food labels, a multivitamin/mineral supplement containing 400 micrograms of folic acid may help keep your heart healthy.

While you're supplementing folic acid, you may also want to add vitamin B_6 and vitamin B_{12} into the mix, Dr. Tucker says. "There's a concern that by taking a lot of folic acid, you can mask a vitamin B_{12} deficiency, a potentially debilitating condition that becomes more common as we age and our bodies stop absorbing vitamin B_{12} as well as they should," she says. In addition, people who have diets low in folic acid also tend to run low in vitamin B_6, another B vitamin that lowers homocysteine levels. So if you're going to supplement one, you might as well supplement all three. Dr. Tucker recommends looking for a multi with up to 10 milligrams of vitamin B_6 and with 6 to 25 micrograms of vitamin B_{12}.

A Multitude of Minerals

Our refined, fast-food diet also leaves us lacking in a couple of essential minerals, says Dr. Tucker—magnesium and calcium. Though it doesn't get a whole lot of press, magnesium has been linked to protection from diabetes, arteriosclerosis, hypertension, some headaches, and osteoporosis (yes, bone loss is a man's problem, too). Yet Americans routinely consume less than the 400 milligrams (the Daily Value) they should each day. And the National Academy of Science's calcium intake recommendations—1,000 milligrams a day for men ages 25 to 65—is a dosage so high that few get enough without supplementation, Dr. Tucker says. As you know, calcium prevents bone loss in your later years, and men lose a significant amount of bone density, too, she says. Taking a multivitamin with 100 milligrams of magnesium and 200 milligrams of calcium (provided you're getting about 800 milligrams from three to four servings of low-fat dairy foods a day) is smart insurance, she says. However, people with heart or kidney problems should not take supplemental magnesium.

Finally, surveys show that zinc may be the mineral most lacking in our diets. That's a serious omission since zinc not only helps keep your immune system strong so that you can fight infections and heal wounds but also is also a main component of your manhood. Zinc helps you produce sperm and maintain healthy semen and testosterone levels. Since you can lose up to 5 milligrams—one-third of the 15-milligram Daily Value—of this sexy mineral with each ejaculation, make sure that you eat enough turkey, oysters, lean beef, or fortified cereals to get what you need each day. Or take a multivitamin/mineral supplement that contains 15 milligrams of zinc. Just don't supplement above that level, according to Dr. Kawachi, or you risk throwing off your body's balance of other important minerals, especially copper, and can lower the body's beneficial high-density lipoprotein cholesterol.

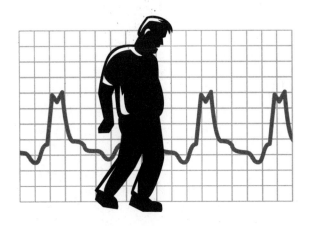

Part Three

Defeating Disease

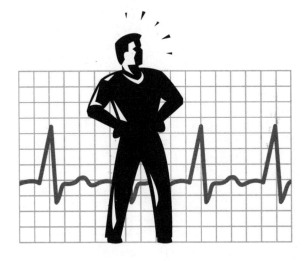

The Disease-Free Lifestyle

Start Living It Tonight

Diseases don't just happen. Something has to go wrong. Most of the time that something has to do with how you treat your body, that is, what you do with it and what you put into it.

In other words, fate is a minor factor in disease. *You* are a major one. If your behavior is in harmony with the way your biochemistry wants to work, you're living a disease-free lifestyle.

So let's get right to it: The major elements of a disease-free lifestyle are a healthy diet, regular physical activity, appropriate body weight, no smoking, controlled stress, and timely medical checkups.

Sense a little déjà vu? None of those six things is what the Pentagon folks would call classified information. We've all heard them since childhood, with overtones of discipline. But "good" behavior isn't the point. The issue's much simpler. Incorporate those six guidelines into your lifestyle and you may prevent disease. Ignore them and you may create disease.

The lifestyle link to disease prevention is so strong that it begs some questions.

Why don't we eat right? In other words, why so much animal fat (an across-the-board disease-causer) and so little fresh fruits and vegetables (risk-reducers for virtually everything)? Because, points out John Wurzelmann, M.D., clinical assistant professor of medicine at the University of North Car-

olina at Chapel Hill School of Medicine, "there really is such a thing as comfort food." Fat, says Dr. Wurzelmann, has a tendency to satisfy you far more than any mere vegetable would. "That's why you enjoy vegetables more when you put a fat dressing on them," he says.

Furthermore, says Moshe Shike, M.D., director of the prevention and wellness program at Memorial Sloan-Kettering Cancer Center in New York City, "it's a habit. You get used to eating hamburgers and french fries, and you don't think about the consequences."

Why don't we exercise? Because we don't need to, according to Walter M. Bortz II, M.D., clinical associate professor of medicine at Stanford University School of Medicine and author of *Dare to Be 100*. Of course, we *do* need to if we want to avoid heart disease, diabetes, and lots of cancers because that's the way our bodies are designed. But it's not the way our everyday life is designed—not when pizzas can be delivered at the touch of a speed dial or home theaters can be controlled at the click of a remote. "In our culture, we don't have to move for anything," Dr. Bortz says. "We're the only species that doesn't have to move even to eat."

Why do we let ourselves get fat? Mostly because we eat too much. "There's no doubt that caloric consumption is too high," Dr. Wurzelmann says. "There are too many fat people in the United States." Obesity is a different risk factor than a lousy diet, but one easily follows from the other.

And inactivity leads to, and follows from, both. "If any other species had food supplied to it the way we do, it would get fat, too," Dr. Bortz says.

Why don't we quit smoking? It's not that a smoker doesn't care that more people die from tobacco use than from automobile accidents, drug abuse, AIDS, and alcohol combined. It's that he's probably addicted. "The nicotine receptors in the brain are very similar to the receptors for cocaine and heroin," says Thomas Glynn, Ph.D., director of cancer science and trends for the American Cancer Society in Atlanta. What's more, those receptors stay eager to receive years after you quit. One puff can get you back to a pack a day before you know it.

Why do we ignore stress? Probably because we're not too sure what it is. "People don't have a lot of knowledge about it and what to do about it," Dr. Shike says. "I think people understand that excess stress has a negative impact on their lives." Heart disease is one negative impact. Undermining the rest of your disease-free lifestyle is another. "Some people, when stressed, run to the refrigerator," Dr. Shike says. "Or they smoke."

Why do we avoid checkups? Denial, according to Dr. Shike, "is the feeling that 'it will never happen to me,' only to somebody else." In reality, all that is being denied is the possibility of early detection, which, for most men-stalking diseases, is the best bet for cure or containment.

Whose Lifestyle Is It Anyway?

By pursuing a disease-free lifestyle, you're doing something about it before it happens. That's a wiser strategy, Dr. Bortz maintains. It's also a major act of heroism, given that you're not exactly smothered with support from the prevailing culture.

Take, for example, the eat-right plank on your disease-free platform. You'll see time and again in the following chapters how much it helps to

Clear the Smoke

Smoking will do in more than internal organs. It takes a pretty heavy hit on health-care budgets, too. A Dutch study figured that health-care costs for smokers can be 40 percent higher than for nonsmokers. So we'd all save a bundle if everybody would just quit smoking, right?

In fact, total health-care costs would actually *rise* in a smokeless society. The reason is obvious: More people would be living longer to run up medical bills in other ways.

But that's not going to happen any time soon. If you're a smoker, you know why: It's hard to quit. It should never be told to a smoker that quitting is easy, says Dr. Thomas Glynn of the American Cancer Society. "But nobody ever said that addiction can't be beat," he says. Here's how.

Really mean it. When it comes to losing the cigarette habit, the road to failure is paved with halfhearted resolve. "Motivation is the absolute determinant," Dr. Glynn says. "Nothing will work unless you woke up that morning and said to yourself, 'This is it. I'm not smoking anymore.' "

Take a walk. Exercise can give you that extra motivational boost and make you feel better while you're trying to quit smoking. "Do something really easy, particularly if you haven't been exercising," Dr. Glynn says. "Take a daily 15-minute walk at a time when you would ordinarily want a cigarette, like in the morning after you've had coffee."

Delay the diet. You really do tend to gain weight as you try to stop smoking, Dr. Glynn says. But his advice is to concentrate on the immediate challenge, which is kicking butts. "A diet is a tough thing to handle at the same time you're quitting smoking," Dr. Glynn says. "Wait until you're safely past the first two or three months of not smoking."

cut down on the animal fat in favor of fiber. But is there enough doctor's advice in the world to offset TV images of Michael Jordan telling you how wonderful it is to eat hamburgers?

"We're a cowboy culture," Dr. Wurzelmann says. "There's a deeply ingrained and continuously reinforced belief that our strength derives from eating cows. What it comes down to is that eating beef is seen as having a lot to do with masculinity."

But that's where taking control of your own lifestyle comes in. Here's how to do it.

Remember what it's all about. The best beginning for a disease-free lifestyle is understanding the end. "You have to know why you're doing it," says Ed Burke, Ph.D., vice president of the National Strength and Conditioning Association in Colorado Springs and co-author of *Getting in Shape*. "If all you want is to lose five pounds to look good when you go to Jamaica on vacation, then don't bother." Instead, Dr. Burke says, think about having more energy always, about feeling stronger forever, about losing weight and keeping it off. "Your approach should be long-term," he says. "Make it part of your life."

Keep things underwhelming. All six disease-free lifestyle elements are essential. But if you suddenly get religion and resolve to change your diet, lose weight, start exercising, and quit smoking on day one, you're going to be overwhelmed. "You can fail miserably if you try to do too much at one time," Dr. Glynn says. "It should be a sequence of lifestyle changes rather than one big one."

The slow-but-sure approach works best for any individual lifestyle element, too. "You can't run a half-hour if you've never walked around the block," Dr. Bortz says. "Take small steps of mastery."

Jungle Story

It could happen to you. You're happily pedaling away on your stationary bike or enjoying the hypnotic pleasure of your daily jog when your thoughts start running toward the meaning of life, the universe, and everything. There's nothing wrong with that in moderation, but it may lead to "the Question"—namely, why exactly is it good for my health to huff and puff for a half-hour every day without necessarily getting anywhere? Why can't you just be healthy effortlessly? It may strike you as bad planning by nature, which has such a grand reputation for design brilliance. What's going on?

Evolution is going on. It's just that it's going on a lot more slowly than human achievement.

"If a man from 5,000 years ago was transported into modern life, physically he'd be exactly the same as us," says Michael Stevenson, Ph.D., a psychologist and sleep specialist at the North Valley Sleep Disorders Center in Mission Hills, California. "Five thousand years is nothing in terms of human evolution. But in that time there has been a tremendous change in what we do."

The disease-free lifestyle, then, bridges the gap

Rewire yourself. For weight loss, gradual and steady progress isn't just easier. It's what works. You didn't gain the weight in two weeks, so you can't lose it healthfully in that amount of time either. You have to learn new behaviors. "Once you got fat, the eating center of your brain became fixed on that," Dr. Bortz says. "If you starve yourself and lose 20 pounds in two weeks, you haven't had time to rewire your brain."

Hence, you haven't accomplished much, and you're probably going to gain the weight back. "Short-term enthusiasm is wonderful, but

between what the human body is designed for and how we actually live these days.

Exercise is a clear example. Aerobics or strength training may be destinationless, but it's not pointless. It puts your behavior in sync with your biology. "For 99.9 percent of our earth time we were very physically active hunter-gatherers, so our whole biology is shaped by movement," says Dr. Walter M. Bortz II of Stanford University School of Medicine. "Only in this last twinkle of biologic time have we become sedentary. And we're paying a heavy price for it."

The same goes for diet. We know that we need to cut down on fat these days, but we have an evolutionary urge to eat it. Why? Because we needed it to store up calories against scarcity back when we had to kill our meat with primitive tools instead of ordering it from a pimply teenager behind a counter. "A guy running around in a loincloth is going to get a lot more calories from eating an animal than from eating an apple," says Dr. John Wurzelmann of the University of North Carolina at Chapel Hill School of Medicine. The problem is that so are we, and we don't need it.

Buried somewhere in that semantic sideshow is a helpful message for the retooling of your lifestyle—namely, that while structured, moderate exercise is best, any kind of regular movement helps. "The major problem is not doing anything," Dr. Stewart says. "With physical activity as the goal, you can build activities into your lifestyle that aren't usually considered exercise—like a sport you think is fun or just mowing the lawn regularly."

Make exercise your cornerstone. The beauty of the disease-free lifestyle is that every element seems to boost every other. For example, reducing stress helps you quit smoking, which helps you exercise, which helps you lose weight. But exercise itself may be the sultan of synergy. "Start by exercising and that will ignite all the other things," Dr. Burke says.

Exercise may work as your lifestyle cornerstone because it has been shown to increase what is known as self-efficacy. "That means that people who exercise have a higher degree of confidence in their ability to do things and they're more likely to do them," Dr. Stewart says. "People who are physically active tend to do other things as well to keep them healthy."

until you get your behavior reprogrammed, your long-term results are going to be poor," Dr. Bortz says.

Get physical. In some circles, it's no longer physically correct to use the term *exercise*. The focus, if you please, is now on *physical activity*. "Exercise tends to be a negative term for many people," says Kerry Stewart, Ed.D., a clinical exercise physiologist and director of cardiac rehabilitation and prevention at Johns Hopkins Bayview Medical Center in Baltimore. "They think of exercise as pain or extremely hard work."

Keep it positive. If you equate a healthy diet with deprivation, you're not going to be very enthusiastic about it. So concentrate on what you should eat, not what you shouldn't, suggests Edward Giovannucci, M.D., Sc.D., assistant professor of medicine at Harvard Medical School. "Rather than obsessing about the fat content of your diet, focus on positive things like getting more whole grains and fruits and vegetables," he says. "Think more along the lines of balance. It's not that you can't eat any dairy products or beef. Just don't make them the focus of your diet."

Heart Disease

Mastering the Man-Killer

Nearly half a million guys die from cardiovascular disease each year—more than the next eight leading causes of death combined.

Scary stuff, right? It doesn't have to be. Quite simply, your cardiovascular system is an amazingly powerful and resilient engineering marvel. Consider the statistics: About the size of two clenched fists, your heart pumps roughly 21,000 gallons of blood a day. In a year, it will beat 3 million times; over 70 years, 2.5 billion times. Stretched end to end, the vessels of your circulatory system—arteries, capillaries, and veins—would measure 60,000 miles. Extremely compact, incredibly reliable, with horsepower to spare. It's like having a Ferrari engine in a Volkswagen Beetle. If you allow yourself to look like a Volkswagen Beetle.

The main point, experts says, is to take care of your heart and it will take care of you. Abuse it and it will still take care of you—for a while. But let's face it, even the finest piece of craftsmanship will succumb to abuse over time.

"What you really have to come to grips with is that what you're putting into your body impacts how your heart and body function. It matters. What you do over the long run matters. How active you are, not one day but over the long run, really matters," says Alice Lichtenstein, D.Sc., spokesperson for the American Heart Association and associate professor at the Jean Meyer USDA Human Nutrition Research Center on Aging at Tufts University in Boston.

Feeding on Fat

Exhibit number one: A high-fat meal at one of those ubiquitous burger stands. Before you can properly wash the grease off your hands—that is, within roughly two hours—much of the fat you've just gobbled down is already in your bloodstream, reducing the natural ability of your arteries to stay open, says Robert DiBianco, M.D., director of cardiology research, the Heart Failure Clinic, and the Risk Factor Reduction Center at Washington Adventist Hospital in Takoma Park, Maryland.

If you infrequently indulge in such a high-fat feast, your liver will eventually clear your blood of that extra fat (also called triglycerides), and all is well. But if this is your standard fare, you have several potential problems. For one thing, women aren't impressed if you're on a first-name basis with the guy at the drive-up window. And for another, you may be on your way to heart disease.

Here's why. Even when we're young, fat, cholesterol, and others bits of bloodstream debris—called plaque—slowly begin to build along the lining of our blood vessels. In most cases, the accumulation is as subtle and gradual as beach erosion.

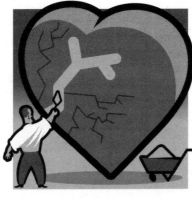

But as the years, Ring Dings, and Buffalo wings go by, plaque from those fattening foods continues to build, especially in areas where your arteries branch, such as those that supply blood to your legs, kidneys, neck, brain, and heart. "The actual physical force of blood on the lining probably damages the lining and allows plaque to form," says Thomas Pickering, M.D., professor of medicine at the Hypertension Center at New York Hospital in Manhattan and author of *Good News about High Blood Pressure*.

And the higher your blood pressure—literally the pressure exerted as blood flows through your vascular system—the greater the damage to its lining (known by the guys with the cold stethoscopes as your endothelium). Further damaging this lining are smoking and diabetes. "When healthy, your endothelium tends to deflect things like platelets and little small packages of fibrin or clot or scar tissue and cholesterol so that, in fact, you don't develop plaque as easily," says Dr. DiBianco. "But damaged endothelium allows these molecules to find their way into the vessel wall. And once they're in the wall, they build up (in the form of plaque) or irritate the blood vessel wall and cause inflammation."

Some guys living the high-fat life won't have seem to have any symptoms until their arteries narrow by about 50 percent. Then things really get ugly. "Clearly, if you have an obstruction to one of the arteries of your heart, anything that increases your need for oxygen—whether it's exercise or emotional upset, intercourse or a meal—will cause angina or chest discomfort," Dr. DiBianco says.

From there, all it takes is one soft plaque to dislodge and clog one of the narrowed arteries to bring on a heart attack. "Although these plaques would make up a minority of plaques in our blood vessels, they're the ones most likely to cause these sudden events that require hospitalization or surgery or can cause death," says Dr. DiBianco.

Impotence: The Other Heart Disease Symptom

If death doesn't scare you enough to make radical changes to protect your heart health, how about a fate some guys might consider worse than death: impotence? We're all too familiar with the grab-your-chest symptoms of heart attack and disease. Less well-known is that the artery supplying blood to the penis is much smaller than those that lead to the heart and, as a result, one of the first to get clogged by fatty plaque.

"What actually happens is that the arterial walls narrow, and so the velocity or the amount of the blood that can move through this artery is decreased," says L. Dean Knoll, M.D., director of research at the Center for Urological Treatment and Research in Nashville. "And when the amount of blood is decreased, you can't fill the spaces in the body of your penis." In fact, one South Carolina study found that erection problems were 80 percent more likely in men with total cholesterol levels above 240 milligrams per deciliter than those with scores below 180 milligrams per deciliter. And while you're watching those numbers, you probably should keep tabs on your blood pressure; hypertension has also been linked to erection problems, says Dr. Knoll.

The Emotional Equation

Most of us know by now that what we eat can kill us, but there are lots of guys who have yet to acknowledge the connection between their emotions and heart disease. Yet some of our most common male emotions—

social isolation, hostility, cynicism, and depression—are almost as devastating to the heart as, say, lunching on lard.

"All of these emotional problems have been found to increase the risk of heart disease and other health problems. And it's not one or the other. In fact, they usually cluster. If you're hostile, you're more likely to have higher levels of depression and you're more likely to be socially isolated," says Redford B. Williams, M.D., professor of psychiatry and director of the Behavioral Medicine Research Center at Duke University Medical Center in Durham, North Carolina, and author of *Lifeskills.*

In fact, if you're a brooding loner, you may be asked to appear in a foreign film someday, but you may not live long enough to see it on the big screen. One five-year study found that people who were socially isolated were three times more likely to die from heart disease than those who had more social lifestyles.

What's more, research has shown that those who already have had heart attacks and were depressed were also more likely to die within six months of their attack, says Dr. Williams. And a Danish study found that those who suffered from despair, low self-esteem, difficulty concentrating, and low motivation were 70 percent more likely to die from heart disease.

"These people weren't clinically depressed, but did have persistent symptoms of depression," says John C. Barefoot, Ph.D., psychologist and associate research professor at Duke University Medical Center in Durham, North Carolina.

What's happening in these situations that increases your risk for heart problems? Anger, frustration, depression, and other emotional upsets are thought to activate your body's fight-or-flight response—an automatic reaction that sets off a chain of internal physiological changes like a home security system gone berserk. Chemicals such as adrenaline

and cortisol, for example, rush to mobilize fat from your body's stores in case you need a high energy source in your bloodstream to fuel your muscles—and your escape, says Dr. Williams. Not surprising, this raises your cholesterol and blood pressure and even makes your blood more likely to clot.

If that's not bad enough, those who are socially isolated, depressed, and hostile seem to have worse health habits, making them more likely to drink and smoke, he says.

Putting the Pieces Together

Hanging around the house in your underwear stinking of cheap booze and cigars, eating artery-clogging fast food, and yelling at the television—not exactly the picture of a man primed to defy death by squeezing every last drop out of life. But as it turns out, neither is focusing solely on improving your emotional outlook or adopting an outlandish cure or two.

"Let's put it this way: You'll never be able to cut open a vitamin E capsule, sprinkle it over a hot-fudge sundae, and not have to worry about the sundae," says Dr. Lichtenstein. To beat heart disease, "you may have to make major fundamental adjustments that become habitual. Accept that taking care of your heart is going to be a lifelong project." But it's really not as difficult as you might think it is. Here's how it's done.

Know your risk. It's true. Some guys have all the luck (thanks for the reminder, Rod Stewart). And some guys have higher risk factors than others. For example, you're at risk for heart disease if a first-degree male relative (like a brother or your dad) under age 55 or a first-degree female relative (like a sister or your mother) under age 65 has suffered a heart attack. If you have both, naturally you're at a higher risk. Got diabetes? High blood pressure? High cholesterol? Low high-density lipoprotein (HDL) cholesterol? Do you smoke?

All six? Your risk is higher still. "Those are your major risk factors, and once you have your cholesterol measured, some kind of decision can be made about just how much risk you have. But you really can't tell until you've had your cholesterol checked," Dr. Lichtenstein says.

Cut your total cholesterol. You've heard it so many times, you're starting to think LDL stands for "lower, dummy, lower." But bear with us. Reducing the "bad" LDL (low-density lipoprotein) cholesterol generated by your diet and raising your "good" HDL cholesterol with exercise can dramatically cut your risk for heart disease. As you probably know, LDL is called the bad cholesterol because it can penetrate artery walls, narrowing vessels and choking off blood. What you may not know is that research has shown that vascular disease patients who cut their total cholesterol by about 20 percent reduced their heart attack risk by two-thirds, says Dr. DiBianco.

"This helped convert soft, vulnerable plaques into more stabilized plaques that are less likely to break off and clog arteries," Dr. DiBianco says. According to the American Heart Association, your goal should be to try to keep your total cholesterol under 200 milligrams per deciliter. Borderline high cholesterol is 200 to 239 milligrams per deciliter, while high cholesterol is over 240 milligrams per deciliter. One of the best ways to lower your cholesterol is to eat less saturated fat, the kind found in meat and dairy products, says Dr. DiBianco.

Bring down your blood pressure. Here are some more numbers that can help add up to a healthy heart and a longer, more active life. When checking your blood pres-

sure—once or twice a year should do—look for a reading of 120/80 millimeters of mercury (pronounce it "120 over 80" just like they do on your favorite hospital drama). That's considered normal. A reading above 140/90 should be of concern. And when your blood pressure is over 160/100, it's definitely too high, says Dr. Pickering. (For more information on beating high blood pressure, see High Blood Pressure on page 92.)

Strong Body, Weak Heart?

They've long been touted as the ultimate test of stamina and, for the less ambitious among us, sanity. But a study by Harvard researchers is raising questions about the effects of triathlons on the hearts of participants.

Sensitive chemical tests performed on participants in the Hawaiian Ironman Triathlon—an event that features a grueling 2.4-mile ocean swim, a 112-mile bike race, and 26.2-mile run—found that the top finishers had elevated levels of proteins usually found in those suffering from a heart attack. Some of the triathletes had abnormal heartbeats, even though none of them showed any sign of heart problems before the race.

"Those participants who pushed themselves the hardest, the top finishers, were the ones that showed the most damage," says a co-author of the study, Nader Rifai, Ph.D., associate professor of pathology at Harvard Medical School and director of clinical chemistry at Children's Hospital in Boston. Obviously, you shouldn't take this as an excuse to blow off regular exercise. But it may just be that too much of a good thing—in this case, strenuous athletic competition—is bad for your heart.

Stop smoking. If you don't want to give up cigarettes for your own heart's sake, do it for your sweetheart's sake. A seven-year study of 353,180 women and 126,500 men who had never smoked found that those who lived with smokers had a roughly 20 percent greater risk of death from heart disease.

Check your road map. We may not like asking for directions, but real guys love to read maps. And by learning to read what Dr. Williams calls your hostility road map, you may very well help save your heart—and your life. "You want to ask yourself three questions when you're in a troubling situation: Is it important? Is my anger justified by the facts? And is there anything I can do to change it? If you get a 'no' answer for any, you try to talk yourself out of being angry," he says. And fewer angry episodes means less deadly stress on your heart.

Make friends with good fats. Here's the good news. You don't have to give up fat. In fact, eating the right kind of fat can actually help your heart. Use olive oil, a source of heart-healthy monounsaturated fat, recommends Alberto Ascherio, M.D., assistant professor of nutrition at the Harvard School of Public Health. "Reducing total fat itself is unlikely to be effective in reducing the risk of coronary disease unless attention is paid to the type of fat," says Dr. Ascherio.

The beneficial effects of a diet high in monounsaturated fat are supported by a landmark study comparing heart disease rates among several European countries and the United States. Researchers poring over the data soon discovered that residents of the Mediterranean country of Crete had the lowest heart disease rate. But Crete also had the highest total fat consumption, with about 40 percent of calories coming from fat—most of it monounsaturated fat from olive oil. Finland ate the most saturated fat and had the highest death rate, Dr. Ascherio says.

Work it out. Sure, 30 minutes of moderately intense aerobic exercise—like jogging, biking, or playing basketball—three times a week will help keep your weight down and your muscles toned. Best of all, it tones the muscle that matters the most: your heart.

"You want your heart in the best shape possible—strong, not flabby—to avoid a heart attack. But even if you did have one, a stronger heart increases your chance of survival," says Howard N. Hodis, M.D., director of the Atherosclerosis Research Unit at the University of Southern California School of Medicine in Los Angeles.

Regular exercise also helps widen blood vessels, increasing blood flow to the heart and helping to remove lesions from your arterial wall, says Dr. Hodis. And if that isn't reason enough to trade your recliner for some running shoes, exercise helps drain anger and reduce blood pressure, both common heartbreakers, he says.

Ask your doctor about aspirin. Research has shown that taking 60 milligrams of aspirin per day—roughly the same amount found in a baby aspirin—can help prevent your first heart attack by making your blood less sticky, Dr. Hodis says. But be careful. Taking too much can have the opposite effect. "A lot of doctors tell their patients to break a regular adult aspirin in half or quarters and take that," Dr. Hodis says. Since taking a daily dose of aspirin has been found to slightly increase your risk for a stroke, talk to your doctor about whether it's right for you.

Examine vitamin E. Dr. Hodis's study shows that vitamin E may benefit the walls of your arteries. For example, his research found that those who took 100 international units or more of vitamin E per day had slower coronary artery lesion progression. Not only that, but the massive four-year Health Professionals Follow-Up Study found that those men who had the highest vitamin E intake—primarily through supplements—had a 40 percent lower risk of coronary disease than the rest of the guys. In addition to making blood less sticky, vitamin E also has what's called an antioxidant effect in arteries. In the same way a coat of primer keeps an iron gate from rusting, antioxidants like vitamin E may protect cholesterol from oxidizing and hardening in arteries.

If you decide to take vitamin E, it should only play a role in your overall strategy for reducing heart disease risk. "You still need to decrease your saturated fat intake, reduce your body weight, and eat lots of fruits and vegetables, your best sources of antioxidant vitamins like C and E," says Dr. Lichtenstein.

Fit in some folic acid and some Bs. Folic acid as well as vitamins B_{12} and B_6 can help reduce levels of an amino acid in the blood called homocysteine that has been found to damage arterial tissue.

"I think there is real promise here," says Ronald M. Krauss, M.D., head of molecular medicine at Lawrence Berkeley National Laboratory at the University of California in Berkeley and chairman of the Nutrition Committee of the American Heart Association. "Although we do not have direct evidence that reducing homocysteine can reduce the risk for heart disease, we strongly recommend that people ensure adequate intakes of folic acid and B vitamins," says Dr. Krauss. Folate (the form of folic acid in foods) is found in fruits such as oranges; in vegetables such as asparagus, beans, and brussels sprouts; and in fortified grains and cereal products. The Daily Value for folic acid is 400 micrograms, and the Daily Value of vitamins B_6 and B_{12} is 2 milligrams and 6 micrograms, respectively, Dr. Krauss says. You may need to take a multivitamin to get that much in a day, however, he adds.

Fill up on fiber. Whether it helps soak up cholesterol or simply prevents you from overeating isn't clear. But the American Heart Association says that getting 25 to 30 grams of fiber a day can cut your risk for heart disease.

"The reasons why are still elusive, but people who eat more fiber have less heart disease," says Dr. Ascherio. One simple way to make sure that you get more fiber in your diet is choosing a breakfast cereal that's high in fiber. Look for brands that provide at least 5 grams of fiber per serving. "Some cereals have surprisingly little fiber, and others are really high. Check the side of the box," he says.

Check your flax. Research has shown that eating bread made with flaxseed may help reduce cholesterol levels. A natural blood thinner, flaxseed apparently helps combat thickening of the blood as we age, says Tom Watkins, Ph.D., laboratory director of the Kenneth Jordan Heart Research Center in Mont Clair, New Jersey.

"Flaxseed oil is rich in alpha-linoleic acid, and in our own studies that appears to be beneficial," says Dr. Ascherio. If you don't have a taste for flaxseed or never bought one of those trendy bread machines, consider munching on a handful of walnuts. "There's increased evidence that walnuts reduce the risk of heart disease because they're also high in alpha-linoleic acid," he says. Found in soybean and corn oil, polyunsaturated fat is much better for your heart than saturated fat.

Trash trans fatty acids. Better living through chemistry? Not always. When food manufacturers wanted to make margarine stiffer and lengthen the shelf life of other products, they created what are called trans fatty acids—a nutritional Frankenstein harder on your heart than even the dreaded saturated fat. "There's no question that trans fatty acids have the worst effect on blood cholesterol," says Dr. Ascherio. "Not only do they increase the bad cholesterol, but also they reduce the good cholesterol, or HDL cholesterol." To purge trans fatty acids from your diet, avoid foods containing partially hydrogenated vegetable oil, suggests Dr. Ascherio. But be vigilant. It's found in prepared foods from bread to frozen french fries.

High Blood Pressure

A Problem with Extra Power

If you're the kind of guy who has all kinds of extra memory on your computer or even a turbocharger on your riding lawn mower, you may be wondering, what's the fuss about high blood pressure? Doesn't higher pressure mean more power? And how in a man's world could that ever be bad?

For one thing, high blood pressure makes you a prime candidate for a stroke, the third leading killer of men. In fact, the National Stroke Association says that between 40 and 90 percent of all stroke victims had high blood pressure before their strokes. "No question about it, high blood pressure leads the hit list," says Ralph Sacco, M.D., director of the Northern Manhattan Stroke Study at Columbia-Presbyterian Medical Center in New York City and spokesperson for the National Stroke Association. What's more, high blood pressure is the leading risk factor for congestive heart failure and has been linked to, among other things, heart disease, kidney disease, and an ominous-sounding problem called brain shrinkage.

If all this sounds fairly negative, you're starting to get the picture. High blood pressure itself may not put you in a pine box—although about 40,000 Americans die from it each year—but it can sure help you along. "We're talking about a problem that affects 50 million people," says Eva Obarzanek, R.D., Ph.D., a research nutritionist at the National Heart, Lung, and Blood Institute in Washington, D.C. "If we could lower people's blood pressure, we could cut the number of serious diseases dramatically."

A peek inside your cardiovascular system shows why.

The Pressure-Plaque Connection

Think of your heart as one incredibly well-built pump and your arteries, veins, and capillaries as a vast plumbing system of flexible, interconnected tubes carrying blood throughout your body. And when we say vast, we mean it: Stretched length-wise, the vessels of your circulatory system would measure an amazing 60,000 miles. In just one day, the average healthy adult heart pumps the equivalent of 2,100 gallons of blood.

The motor behind that movement is your heartbeat. For purposes of measuring the force your heart exerts, experts divide your heartbeat into two phases. When blood is squeezed out of your heart, that's called your systolic pressure—the first number in your blood pressure equation. When your heart relaxes and refills with blood, that's called diastolic pressure, the second number. A reading of 120/80 millimeters of mercury (120 over 80) is considered normal. Experts say that a reading above 140/90 should be of concern. And when your blood pressure is higher than 160/100, it's definitely a problem, says Dr. Thomas Pickering of the Hypertension Center at New York Hospital.

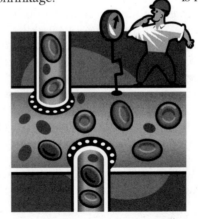

Here's where it gets weird. When that pressure rises higher than normal, the ever-protective lining of your arteries, called the endothelium, can't keep plaque and other bits of blood debris from entering the vessel wall. The result: Before long, plaque starts to build up, clogging your arteries and blood vessels, says Dr. Robert DiBianco of Washington Adventist Hospital.

High blood pressure also strains your heart. Given the right stress—say, running or some other form of aerobic exercise—your heart will grow so that it can pump more blood. Not so when you have high blood pressure. Instead, your heart just gets thicker, which down the road can cause your heart to outgrow its blood supply. And this makes it more susceptible to narrowing of the arteries that supply blood to the heart, Dr. Pickering says.

Driving It Down

The good news is that there's plenty you can do to beat high blood pressure. And while you're on the way, you can have the satisfaction of knowing that you'll be defying heart disease and stroke as well. In fact, researchers poring over data from the famed Framingham Heart Study have found that the combination of lower cholesterol levels, lower blood pressure, and a decline in cigarette smoking can dramatically reduce heart disease deaths. Here's how.

Make a DASH for it. Even if you don't already have high blood pressure, the results of a study called Dietary Approaches to Stop Hypertension (DASH) may make you want to run to your nearby produce stand. The 11-week study compared three diets: a standard high-fat American diet, which was the control diet; a diet high in fruits and vegetables; and a "combination diet" that was low in saturated fat, total fat, and cholesterol, and high in fruits, vegetables, and low-fat dairy products. When it was over, the average blood pressure for the combination diet group was 5.5 millimeters of mercury systolic and 3.0 millimeters of mercury diastolic lower than the control diet group. Among those with high blood pressure, the combination diet group's average blood pressure was 11.4 millimeters of mercury systolic and 5.5 millimeters of mercury diastolic lower than the control diet group's.

A typical day of eating from the combination platter? It consists of 7 to 8 servings of grains (as in bread or cereal); 4 to 5 servings of vegetables; 4 to 5 servings of fruits; 2 to 3 dairy products; up to 2 servings of meat, poultry, or fish; and 2½ servings of fat and oils (the equivalent of 2½ teaspoons of oil).

Strive for fitness. Research has also shown that the fittest guys have the lowest blood pressures and cholesterol levels. And when followed over many years, the rate of death from cardiovascular disease is higher in the least fit than in the most fit. Thirty minutes of aerobic exercise at least three times a week is a good start. And add some weight training to the mix when you're ready for more, suggests Dr. Pickering.

Pick up the pace. If you're a runner concerned about high blood pressure, you may want to pick up the pace. Researchers from the National Runners Health Study discovered that running faster had a 13.3 times' greater impact on lowering blood pressure than a leisurely jog. The researchers noted that "the principle should apply to any sustained and vigorous exercise, such as cycling and swimming."

Tame your tongue. Does talking fast raise blood pressure? Researchers measured the blood pressures and heart rates of 111 cardiac patients as they read the U.S. Constitution rapidly for two minutes, then slowly for two minutes. Rapid reading triggered a rise in the subjects' blood pressures and heart rates, according to the study. Never forget: You have the right to remain silent.

Shake the salt. Not all the experts agree, but for now it's probably a good idea to limit salt intake to help shake high blood pressure. It may just bring it down a few points or even prevent it. The American Heart Association recommends eating no more than 6 grams of salt a day. In case you've never counted, a teaspoon of salt is about 6 grams. But when tracking your salt intake, keep in mind that lots of prepared foods contain massive amounts of added salt.

Cancer

Playing the Prevent Defense

Let's all admit it: Cancer's scary. It's the very symbol of death by disease. It has had its way for most of the century.

But times have changed, and so should our attitudes—in this case, from cowering fatalism to bold confrontation. "You don't have to be cancer's victim," says Dr. John Wurzelmann of the University of North Carolina at Chapel Hill School of Medicine. "And you don't need to be afraid to think about it. There really is a lot of reason to be optimistic."

To be sure, cancer is still a scourge, still the number two cause of death in the United States. Three of the four most common and fatal cancers (colorectal, prostate, and lung) affect men most often. What's more, almost all cancers attack and kill men at higher rates than women.

But here's the rest of the picture. People are surviving almost all kinds of cancer more than they ever did before. Early-detection techniques are better, so more cancerous tissue is being removed before it spreads. Treatment options have expanded.

It's not just the doctors who got smarter. The rest of us are learning that there are a whole lot of things we can do—or stop doing—to keep cancer away in the first place. We're taking control. As a team of Harvard-affiliated researchers put it in the Harvard Report on Cancer Prevention, "Cancer is indeed a preventable illness."

Beating the Bad Cells

Cancer is bad cells, pure and simple. Something goes

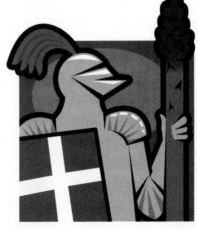

wrong with the DNA, and eventually, a fast-growing collection of toxin-spewing, energy-absorbing, organ-destroying cells have begun to take over some part of your body. It can start just about anywhere, from your brain to your testicles, and end up just about anywhere else. Once cancer starts to migrate from its place of birth (a process known as metastasis), it's hard to treat.

Your mission is to keep all that stuff from happening. Some of the risk factors, such as heredity and age, are out of your hands. But—and hear this well—most are not. Nearly two-thirds of cancer deaths in the United States are caused by factors entirely within your control. And guess what? Those controllable factors are none other than the usual suspects—smoking, a lousy diet, and a lack of exercise.

Studies have shown fairly clearly that obese men run a higher risk of at least colorectal and prostate cancer. Know that about 31 percent of American men are overweight (that is, 20 or more percent above their ideal weight) and you start to get the picture. What's more, the extra pounds may affect men more than women, probably because men tend to carry the fat in their abdomen, where it's more biologically active.

One way you get fat is by eating fat, especially animal fat. Not only does fat intake put you on the fast track to obesity but also there are strong indications that foods high in animal fat, such as dairy foods and red meat, increase your risk for a number of cancers, including prostate, colorectal, and even nonmelanoma skin cancer.

Another way you get fat is through inactivity. It's also another way you get cancer, especially colorectal cancer

Now to smoking. What don't you already know about smoking's sinister deeds? How about this: Smoking causes a whopping 30 percent of all cancer mortality, but not only because it's responsible for more than 90 percent of lung cancer deaths. If you smoke, you also increase your risk for oral, esophagus, pancreas, larynx, bladder, and kidney cancers. And there's newer evidence linking it to prostate and colon cancer, the latter in a special way. "Smoking seems to be an 'early' risk factor for colon cancer," says Dr. Edward Giovannucci of Harvard Medical School. "If you're smoking at age 20, that may not show up as a risk factor for colon cancer until age 60 or 70, whether you quit or not."

So smoking, eating junk food, getting fat, and being lazy aren't merely abstractions that are "bad for your health," whatever that means. They can cause cancer. Put another way, not smoking, eating well, staying trim, and exercising are real things you can do to help prevent cancer. Here's how to make those real things a real part of your life.

Listen to your mom. Mama put it this way: "You eat your vegetables now, young man." The National Cancer Institute puts it this way: "Populations consuming diets high in fruits and vegetables tend to have a lower cancer risk." They both mean the same thing, so do what Mama said. The National Cancer Institute suggests eating five or more servings of fruits and vegetables a day. More is better, according to Dr. Giovannucci, and variety is also important. He suggests that you eat, among other things, leafy green vegetables, deeply colored orange vegetables like carrots, tomatoes, garlic and onions, broccoli, and citrus fruits.

Listen to Neil Young. Excuse the apparent redundancy, but there's another reason for pinching your overall calorie count besides losing weight. It has to do with the damages of oxidation. "It's the 'Rust Never Sleeps' theory of cancer," Dr. Wurzelmann says. "We're under a lot of oxidative stress. The more we eat, the more the furnace burns and the more likely it is we're going to create something that causes cancer. We can reduce that oxidative stress by reducing our total caloric intake."

Hide the beef. Studies consistently show that colon cancer is low wherever meat consumption is low. There is some suggestion that increased meat consumption could also increase the risk for prostate cancer. Vegetarians, even in the United States, have a lower risk of cancer than their carnivorous compatriots. "Try to stay as close to a vegetarian diet as you can," advises William J. Catalona, M.D., chief of urologic surgery at Washington University School of Medicine in St. Louis. "If you do want to eat meat, try to emphasize fish and chicken and limit the amount of red meat that you eat—ideally, not more than one serving per week."

Iron out your risk. Dr. Wurzelmann led a study that showed a connection between high levels of iron and cancer. For the most part, he says, the link is a corollary of the red meat problem. "If you eat beef, you eat iron," Dr. Wurzelmann says. But, he adds, there does seem to be a clear connection between iron overload itself and liver cancer. "People who are supplementing with iron might not be doing themselves a favor," he says. "I think this medical practice deserves serious reappraisal."

Get enough selenium. Research has pointed to a "very promising" (Dr. Giovannucci's words) role for the trace mineral selenium in reducing the risk of several cancers, including prostate and colorectal.

"There's more work to do," Dr. Giovannucci says. "But at this point it might be a reasonable thing to take selenium supplements given our current knowledge. More research is necessary to make firm recommendations, though." The Daily Value for selenium is 70 micrograms.

Go for the grape. The revered grape has long been a folk cure, but a 1997 study by University of Illinois at Chicago researchers has put some scientific muscle behind the idea. The preliminary evidence in test tubes and animals is that resveratrol, a compound found in grapes and other plants, may slow down tumor growth, block the action of cancer-causing agents, and even clean up precancerous cells.

Yes, there's resveratrol in wine, but Varro E. Tyler, Ph.D., dean emeritus of Purdue University School of Pharmacy and Pharmacal Sciences in West Lafayette, Indiana, and distinguished professor emeritus of pharmacognosy (natural pharmaceuticals), suggests taking advantage of the potential benefits by adding some real grapes or a glass of grape juice to your diet.

Smother it with onions. If you're in the habit of saying "hold the onions," you might reconsider. Dutch researchers found that volunteers who ate half an onion a day had half the risk of stomach cancer that their sweeter-breath co-subjects did. The heroes in onions are allylic sulfides, which help enzymes neutralize cancer-causing substances.

Get enough vitamin C. It's always a controversial topic, but when researchers look into the health role of vitamin C, they usually find that it protects against certain cancers, according to the National Cancer Institute. The best evidence is that it fights cancers of the esophagus, mouth, and stomach. But it also helps fend off pancreas and rectum cancers.

Protecting the Prostate

Prostate cancer is to men roughly what breast cancer is to women. Each is far and away the most prevalent cancer for its respective sex, and each is a solid second (behind lung cancer) in deaths caused. And just as its breast-based relative was for women, prostate cancer has become the emblem of middle-age male health angst. It seems like that plum-size gland is going to get you, sooner or later.

But doctors have noticed that men are taking another tip from women. They're fighting back. Proof? Well, how often did you

Blowing Smoke

Dr. Thomas Glynn of the American Cancer Society has a lot to say about lung cancer, and it doesn't take long for him to say it. Here's a transcript of a lecture he sometimes gives: "This is going to be easy. Don't smoke. Thank you for listening."

Smokers sometimes give themselves little talks, too: statements meant to make them and their loved ones think that they'll somehow be able to smoke and not hurt themselves. Here are some of the most common—and error-ridden.

"I'll stop when I'm older." True, quitting smoking reduces your risk whenever you do it, but sooner is much better than later. In the words of the American Lung Association, "The more you smoke and the longer you smoke, the greater your risk of lung cancer."

"I'll get lots of antioxidants." It was once thought that antioxidants like beta-carotene reduced lung cancer risk. But it's a false friend, as several studies have shown. "Beta-carotene was actually found to be a culprit in the progression of lung cancer," says Dr. Warren Heston of the Memorial Sloan-Kettering Cancer Center. And, he adds, so may single supplements, such as lycopene. So much for that one.

"I'll eat lots of vegetables." They help, but there's no salad bar big enough to offset the smoking risk. As a team of Harvard-affiliated researchers put it in a 1996 report on cancer prevention, "A smoker consuming the largest tolerable amounts of vegetables is still at much higher risk of lung cancer than a nonsmoker."

"The smog is going to get me anyway." Says who? "It's really difficult to pin lung cancer on air pollution,"

hear prostate cancer or the prostate itself even mentioned 15 years ago?

"Prostate cancer has come out of the closet," Dr. Catalona says. "Everybody knows

says Bill McDonnell, M.D., Ph.D., a medical officer for the U.S. Environmental Protection Agency (EPA) in Chapel Hill, North Carolina. "There's just not very strong evidence for that." And even if there were, Dr. McDonnell points out, "cigarette smoking is in a class by itself, both in regard to the variety and amount of inhaled substances and with regard to its ability to cause cancer."

"I'll avoid other carcinogens." Indeed, there are some to avoid, most notably radon, which the EPA estimates is found at higher-than-acceptable levels in 1 out of 15 homes in the United States. On-the-job exposure to things such as asbestos, uranium, arsenic, and certain petroleum products is also something to look out for. But all of them are more dangerous when combined with smoking. And remember, another environmental hazard that causes the death of some 3,000 nonsmokers a year from lung cancer, according to the EPA, is none other than tobacco smoke—from other people's cigarettes.

"I'll catch it early." That's a good strategy for most cancers but usually hopeless for lung cancer. "By the time it's detectable, it's generally too late to do anything," Dr. Glynn says. "If you go in for a chest x-ray and they find a tumor, the outlook's not good."

"Lots of people beat it." But most don't. Lung cancer's five-year survival rate is 13 percent, one of the lowest of all cancers. "It's a virtually certain killer," Dr. Glynn says. "You're looking at a one in eight chance that you're going to be alive in five years. And most people from the time of diagnosis are dead in two years."

For the record, your prostate gland surrounds the urethra at the base of your penis and helps produce the semen you're so fond of giving away. It seems to be built to go partially wrong. It often starts to enlarge (benignly) in your forties, and from 30 percent to 50 percent of men in their forties and fifties have precancerous lesions on its surface. Not all develop into cancer, but those that do are, on average, diagnosed at age 72. But with new methods of detection, the age at diagnosis is decreasing.

You don't have to die from prostate cancer. "The disease is definitely treatable," says Warren Heston, Ph.D., director of the George M. O'Brien Urology Research Center at the Memorial Sloan-Kettering Cancer Center in New York City. "Early detection is very much a big key."

But your best weapon against prostate cancer is not getting it in the first place. And, hey, most guys don't. "About one in five men are diagnosed with prostate cancer in their lifetime," Dr. Catalona estimates. "So the chances are 80 percent that you won't be."

Not the worst of odds. And you can make them better by adding the following prostate-specific weapons to your anti-cancer arsenal.

Whip up some spaghetti. Vegetables, in general, fight cancer. But it's tomatoes that go right after prostate cancer, according to Dr. Giovannucci, who worked on the Harvard study that came up with this happy news. Tomatoes are rich in the antioxidant lycopene, which may lower risk of prostate cancer. "For prostate cancer, it's important to include tomatoes in your diet—tomato sauce, in particular," Dr. Giovannucci says. He suggests two one-cup servings a week.

what a breast is, and everybody knows what a lung is. But until very recently a lot of men didn't know what a prostate was, or where it was."

Grab some soy, boy. Soy products are rich in genistein, a weak estrogen with antioxidant properties that, studies have shown, will slow the progression of prostate cancer. That may explain the fact that Japanese men eat a lot of soy and seldom get prostate cancer, while American men eat almost no soy and get lots of prostate cancer.

Get enough vitamin E. Dr. Heston points to a Finnish study that found that those who took 50 milligrams of vitamin E "actually had a 30 percent reduction in the development of full prostate cancer." Dr. Heston suggests that getting your Daily Value of 30 international units, or about 20 milligrams, would be beneficial.

Colorectal Concerns

No site is very pleasing for a tumor, but the notion of a cancer taking up residence in your bowel is extra queasy. Why, of all places, is it there?

For one thing, this is a place with a high cell turnover rate, so the likelihood of cancer developing is increased. Another reason is that the colon is full of bacteria that produce carcinogens. Cancers in either of those two bowel parts are usually lumped into the "colorectal" category. About 54,900 deaths from colorectal cancer were predicted for 1997, about 10 percent of all cancer deaths.

But actually, people are getting less colorectal cancer these days. The total incidences dropped from about 149,000 new cases in 1994 to an estimated 131,200 cases in 1997. This may be due to adopting healthier lifestyles, says Dr. Wurzelmann.

Early detection and removal of precancerous polyps are also likely playing a role. "I'm not seeing the big, bulky, extensive cancers that I used to 15 or 20 years ago," and the reason is early detection, says Bruce Wolff, M.D., professor of surgery at the Mayo Clinic and Mayo Foundation in Rochester, Minnesota, and a member of the American Society of Colon and Rectal Surgeons.

If you want to increase your odds that there won't be anything to detect—early or later—doctors recommend taking these steps.

Ask for aspirin. Popping a baby aspirin once a day seems to help with a lot of things, including colorectal cancer. According to Dr. Wurzelmann, aspirin increases the rate at which cancer cells kill themselves off. Some doctors are reasonably concerned about stomach bleeding or discomfort from daily aspirin doses. But, says Dr. Wurzelmann, "if you can tolerate aspirin, it may be a reasonable way to prevent cancer. Further research is needed, however, before final recommendations can be made." Check with your doctor before you start popping aspirin.

Cool it with the booze. Heavy drinking has been connected with esophageal cancer, but it also increases the likelihood of the polyps that are precursors to colorectal cancer. "People who drink a lot can get more polyps," Dr. Wurzelmann says. "Several different studies support that connection."

Bulk up with fiber. The verdict is in on high-fiber diets, and it's a good one for colorectal cancer prevention. Canadian researchers, looking at 13 studies involving more than 15,000 people, found that adding 13 grams of fiber a day to your diet could reduce your risk by 31 percent. The National Cancer Institute suggests that you increase your fiber intake to between 20 and 30 grams a day.

Embrace brassicas. For colorectal cancer, there is convincing proof that vegetables decrease risk. It's a kid's nightmare. Eat lots of different vegetables but be sure to include broccoli, brussels sprouts, cabbage, and cauliflower. All are members of the brassica vegetable family, and they could be a grown-up guy's salvation. They contain chemicals that appear to reduce the risk of colorectal cancer. "Eat as much as you can enjoy," suggests Dr. Wurzelmann.

Do calisthenics for your colon. One of the more proven ways to reduce colon cancer is to get moving. No, not *that* kind of moving. We're talking physical activity here—

exercise. The Centers for Disease Control and Prevention and the American College of Sports Medicine recommend 30 minutes of moderate exercise daily. Even if that exercise is divided into 10-minute segments, it's enough to reduce the risk of colon cancer.

Saving Your Skin

And then there's the fastest-rising cancer of all. Malignant melanoma—the deadly variety of skin cancer—is increasing so rapidly that its death toll keeps going up even though the survival rate is actually getting better. In addition, nonmelanoma skin cancer—basal and squamous cell carcinoma—is the most common cancer among U.S. Whites.

The sun is to blame. And the fact is that we've been spending a lot more time under it in recent decades. The great outdoors is a wonderful place to be, but not if you don't protect your skin from the sun. And the lighter your skin, the more at risk you are.

Still, skin cancer is one of the more treatable cancers since the problem is usually right on the surface. It's also preventable. Here's what you can do in addition to reducing the amount of fat in your diet.

Cover up. It's a sunny day and the mercury's rising. Perfect for cutoffs and a tank top, right? Not if you want to protect yourself from skin cancer. "If you're going out in the sunlight, wear protective clothing," says John E. Wolf Jr., M.D., chairman of the department of dermatology at Baylor College of Medicine in Houston. "That means a long-sleeve shirt and long pants. If you have thinning hair, it's particularly important that you wear a hat or a cap."

Rub on the sunscreen. Not just for a day on the beach but for all day every day. "The biggest mistake people make is thinking that they only have to wear a sunscreen when they're sitting at a ball game or playing tennis," Dr. Wolf says. "The ideal way to do it is to put the sunscreen on as part of your regular morning routine."

Gloomy weather is no exception. "As a matter of fact, cloudy days are perhaps more dangerous than sunny days because people don't think about protecting themselves," Dr. Wolf says. "But 70 percent of the rays are coming through."

Reapply if you're out for a long exposure or you get wet. And make sure that your sunscreen is strong enough. A sun protection factor (SPF) of 15 is usually sufficient, according to Dr. Wolf. But bump it up as high as 45 if your skin is extra-fair, if you burn easily, or if you're taking diuretics or antibiotics.

Stay out of the midday sun. "Use common sense about when you're out," Dr. Wolf says. "The most intense rays are generally between 10:00 A.M. and 3:00 P.M., so the best time to exercise or mow the lawn would be before or after that time."

Find a better status symbol. Other than the chief executive officer suntan, that is. "All a suntan is is your skin's desperate attempt to protect itself from sunlight," Dr. Wolf says. "It's not healthy." Neither are tanning booths. "The rays used in tanning parlors are less likely to burn you, but they can do all the other nasty things," Dr. Wolf says.

Take a look. Dr. Wolf suggests examining your own skin monthly, with the help of a mirror or a willing accomplice. Any noticeable change is worth a visit to a dermatologist. That includes moles. "Having a lot of moles is a risk factor for melanoma," he says. According to the American Cancer Society, the key warning signs of nonmelanoma cancer are a new growth, a spot that is enlarging, or a sore that does not heal within three months. Moles that grow, change continuously, or have the American Cancer Society's A, B, C, D characteristics merit a trip to a physician who can evaluate skin diseases.

A: It is asymmetrical; the halves don't match.
B: Its border is irregular.
C: The color is not uniformly black or brown and may have patches of blue, red, and white.
D: The diameter is greater than 6 millimeters.

Stroke

*Defending Against
"Brain Attack"*

Most of us are infinitely more familiar with the symptoms of a Big Mac attack than a brain attack, also known as a stroke. In fact, one study found that 27 percent of the general public didn't know a single warning sign of stroke, whereas the craving for beef, though hard to describe, often ends with a visit to your favorite grease pit.

If you want to be a card-carrying death defier, it's imperative that you bone up your knowledge about stroke—the nation's third leading killer. The brain cells and life you save could be your own. "The majority of stroke sufferers do not get to the hospital within the three-hour time frame we need to help them," says Fletcher McDowell, M.D., professor of neurology at Cornell University Medical College in New York City and president of the Burke Medical Research Group in White Plains, New York. "If you get treatment within that time period, medication may reverse the stroke process or limit its extent."

Part of the problem is that some consider stroke an old person's disease. Guess again. While most stroke victims are over age 65, nearly 30 percent are under 65. "It can happen at any age," says LaRoy Penix, M.D., assistant professor of neurology at the University of Kentucky College of Medicine in Lexington, and faculty associate at the Sanders-Brown stroke program, also at the university. "We have a child here now who had a stroke at the age of 12."

The Center of the Stroke

The brain of a stroke victim tells the story. In the most common scenario, an ischemic stroke, an artery leading to the brain has been blocked by a blood clot. Whether blood flow is blocked by a clot or fatty plaque—the same mixture of cholesterol and other debris that can cause heart attacks—the result is the same. Starved of blood, oxygen, and other vital nutrients for even a few minutes, brain cells begin to die, Dr. McDowell says.

When this occurs you're likely to get some signs that something is seriously wrong: sudden loss of vision in one eye; weakness, numbness, or tingling on one side of the body; difficulty speaking or understanding what people are saying; trouble walking; severe dizziness; or unsteadiness. It's a list you'll want to remember: One study found that 52 percent of stroke patients were unaware they were experiencing a stroke.

"These may be warning signs that the circulation in the brain is not working right and you are at risk for stroke and should seek medical attention," says Dr. Ralph Sacco of the National Stroke Association.

The sooner you seek it, the better. Statistics show that most stroke victims don't report to an emergency room until more than 24 hours after their first symptoms—many hours too late for the best possible treatment. Make it in time and chances are good that the

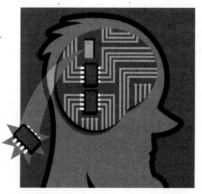

doctors will give you what's called a clot-buster to try to dissolve the blockage and get the blood flowing again, Dr. Sacco says.

If blood flow isn't restored, entire regions of your brain can die. And since these different regions are responsible for various bodily functions— memory, vision, and so on—the shutdown results in familiar forms of disability. Someone who suffers a small stroke, for example, might temporarily lose the use of the muscles in one side of his face. More widespread damage to a key area of the brain can have even more devastating results. "If the area controlling motor function is damaged, for example, that can cause paralysis. Or if that area controls vision, then there's vision loss," Dr. Sacco says.

What, you may ask, are the main culprits in this debilitating, and often deadly, scenario? In addition to plaque buildup or clots, often it's years of high blood pressure—literally the pressure caused by blood on arterial walls—that cause "hardening of the arteries to the brain, small-vessel clogging, or particles blocking arteries," Dr. Sacco says. In fact, high blood pressure is the single most important controllable stroke risk factor. And, of course, anything that helps keep your arteries and blood vessels clear—such as eating less saturated fat and more fiber, losing weight, and lowering your cholesterol—will go a long way in helping you avoid not only stroke but heart disease as well. In fact, reducing your risk for heart disease will also reduce your likelihood of a stroke. (For more information on these strategies, see Heart Disease on page 86.)

Going on the Attack

Don't wait for a stroke before you swing into action. In addition to quitting smoking (another huge risk factor), there are several ways you can fight back against brain attack.

Get a neck check. If any of those stroke symptoms sound vaguely familiar, visit your doctor and have him warm up his stethoscope. But after he checks your chest—heart disease, you know—ask him to listen for a bruit (BREW-ee) in your neck. When the carotid arteries on either side of your neck are narrowed by plaque, they make a rushing sound doctors call a bruit.

"It's not foolproof, but when a general practitioner suspects stroke, he'll perform one

of these. If he doesn't like what he hears, he'll send you to a neurologist for a closer look," says Dr. Penix.

Bring down your blood pressure. Since guys who have high blood pressure before age 45 are 10 times more likely to suffer a stroke later in life, it's vital that you bring yours down. "Regular aerobic exercise and weight loss are two of the best ways to begin to lower your blood pressure," says Dr. Sacco. Try to get 30 minutes of moderate aerobic exercise at least three times a week. Here are the numbers to shoot for: A reading of 120/80 millimeters of mercury (pronounced 120 over 80) is considered normal. Experts say a reading above 140/90 should be of concern. And when your blood pressure is higher than 160/100, it's definitely too high.

Play anyway. You don't need to be diagnosed with high blood pressure to get active, but you can still cut your stroke risk. The Northern Manhattan Stroke Study at Columbia-Presbyterian Medical Center in New York City found that the risk of stroke is 2½ times greater among people who do not exercise. "What impressed us was discovering just how little exercise it took to get these spectacular benefits," Dr. Sacco says. People who walked 20 minutes three times a week were 57 percent less likely to suffer a stroke. Exercise such as bicycling, swimming, hiking, and tennis reduced stroke risk by nearly two-thirds.

Take a sip—occasionally. Alcohol can increase or decrease your stroke risk, depending on how much you drink. In this same study, occasional-to-moderate drinkers who consumed from one alcoholic drink a month to two drinks a day had a 50 percent lower risk than nondrinkers, according to Dr. Sacco. Alcohol—even grape juice, if you abstain from drinking—is thought to make blood less sticky, reducing the risk of clotting and increasing the "good" cholesterol. But don't take this as a license to binge. Drinking more than two drinks per day raises your stroke risk and leads to other health problems.

Pneumonia

The Strong Will Survive

Pneumonia's a bully. It picks on the very young, the old, and the weak. But like most bullies, it'll back off if you stand up to it.

Taking it seriously is a good first step. If you've written off pneumonia as a has-been of a disease, write it back on. Granted, the advent of antibiotics dethroned it from its pre-1936 status as the nation's top cause of death. But there's a lot of fight left in this old killer. Teaming up with influenza, it's still the sixth leading cause of death in the United States. And the number of pneumonia-caused deaths has actually been on the rise, from less than 55,000 in 1980 to more than 80,000 in 1995.

Pneumonia usually swoops in for the kill after some other disease—say, diabetes, chemotherapy-treated cancer, or heart disease—has weakened you. "Even many who die from 'old age' really die of pneumonia," says Ronald Greeno, M.D., co-director of respiratory therapy and pulmonary function at Good Samaritan Hospital in Los Angeles.

Pneumonia is what they call an infectious pulmonary disease, caused usually either by viruses or (much more seriously) bacteria that overpower your lung's defenses and take over. Pretty soon, oxygen isn't getting to your blood the way it should and your cells aren't working right. That can be fatal.

And while the majority of deaths from flu-derived pneumonia in our antibiotic era are in people over 65, that's by no means all of them. "The most common bacterial pneumonia— pneumococcal pneumonia, also known as *Streptococcus pneumoniae*—very often follows a

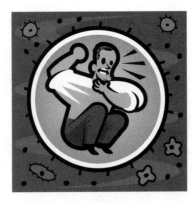

bout of influenza at any age," says Alfred Munzer, M.D., a pulmonologist at Washington Adventist Hospital in Takoma Park, Maryland, and past president of the American Lung Association. "It is much more likely to be fatal in people who are debilitated or elderly, but it certainly can also be fatal in younger people."

Watching Your Viral Signs

What hits younger and middle-age men a lot more often than bacterial pneumonia is either viral pneumonia or pneumonia caused by mycoplasmas, which are bugs falling somewhere in between a virus and bacterium. Since these types are rarely lethal and usually won't land you in the hospital, you hear them referred to as walking pneumonia. Walking is about as much as you'll feel like doing if you have it.

"You can recognize somebody with viral pneumonia because they usually have a dry, hacking, nonproductive cough combined with a fever," says Dr. Munzer.

So if you don't want to be the guy doing the coughing, do your best to follow these tips.

Know the symptoms. Doctors can usually knock out bacterial pneumonia with antibiotics, but not if you don't seek treatment. The problem is that the symptoms are often a lot like flu symptoms—fever, cough, chest pains, phlegm.

Another red flag is a cough that comes in violent attacks, which can signal mycoplasma pneumonia. And, says Dr. Munzer, "if you're bringing up a lot of phlegm and you have a fever, with chest pains that are aggravated by breathing, then you have to start thinking seriously about pneumonia."

Seek treatment pronto. As with most diseases, early diagnosis and treatment speed your recovery of pneumonia. Getting doctor-shy because you simply assume that you have a bad flu—or the more common and less dangerous viral pneumonia—is a dubious piece of self-diagnosis, according to Dr. Greeno.

Besides, adds Steven Mostow, M.D., professor of medicine at the University of Colorado in Denver and chairman of the American Thoracic Society's Committee on the Prevention of Pneumonia and Influenza, in New York City, "there are therapies with any number of compounds that will shorten mycoplasma disease dramatically. And you'll feel a hell of a lot better much more quickly."

Get vaccinated. Yes, there's a pneumonia vaccine. And while it won't fend off every type of pneumonia in existence, it will protect you from the most common bacterial pneumonia, pneumococcal. It's relatively cheap (about $25), it's covered by Medicare, it's side effect–free, and it will last you at least 10 years, perhaps a lifetime. And still, sighs Dr. Munzer, "it's probably the most underutilized of all the vaccines."

Dr. Munzer adds, "there's no harm in *anybody* who's interested in preventive medicine asking his doctor about taking the vaccine. If you want to take it, you should be encouraged to do so."

Get a flu shot. The logic is simple. Influenza can lead to pneumonia. So don't get influenza. "There's one way to avoid the flu, and that's to get an annual flu shot," Dr. Mostow says. "I recommend it even for young, healthy men."

Take your time. If you rush your recovery, you run the risk of a relapse. Remember, it takes longer to recover at age 45 than it does at age 25. And some walking pneu-

monias, such as mycoplasma, leave you weak for many weeks. Rest, after all, is the cure for walking pneumonia, says Dr. Munzer. So stop walking. Take a load off.

Science 1, Mom 1

"Don't go out in that cold without a jacket. You'll catch pneumonia." Mom had your health in mind when she told you that (and told you, and told you, and told you). But, sorry to tell you at this late date, she was misinformed, at least about the pneumonia angle. "Your mother was wrong about that," says Dr. Steven Mostow of the University of Colorado. "Cold air has nothing to do with your immune system being depressed."

Dr. Mostow knows whereof he speaks. He was part of a team of researchers whose mission it was to verify (or debunk) old wives' tales. In the noble pursuit of medical truth, they turned fire hoses on volunteers in bathing suits out on the Runnymeade Plain in England—and you don't have to be an expert in Old World geography to know that that's pretty darn cold. While the soaked subjects were left outside to shiver, the control group was watching television in warm huts.

"There was no difference between the two groups in the incidence or the severity of either colds or flu or pneumonia," Dr. Mostow says.

But the wives'-tale patrol also came up with another surprising finding. They made a three-way comparison among acetaminophen (Tylenol), vitamin C, and chicken soup in the treatment of influenza. Chicken soup won. "Something in chicken soup actually hastens recovery from the flu," Dr. Mostow says. "But it has never been isolated. There's a Nobel Prize lurking in chicken soup."

Your mom could have told them that.

HIV and AIDS

Turning the Corner on a Killer

Remember 10, maybe 15 years ago, when AIDS was an issue as much as an illness? Remember how confusing and controversial it was? It seemed like sometimes we'd forget it was a real disease that was really killing people.

Nowadays, we're more realistic, not to mention optimistic. We've learned how to avoid getting AIDS, and doctors are learning how to keep people from dying of it. In fact, the news about AIDS has been so good lately that, well, it seems like sometimes we forget that it's a real disease that's really killing people.

Okay, so complacency's unwise, as AIDS researchers go out of their way to point out. Duly noted. But there's also no denying that the spirit of the thing has changed for the better. There's less trembling and more treating. What felt like a mandatory death sentence has been lifted somewhat.

The statistics back up the optimism. Simply put, fewer Americans are getting AIDS, and fewer are dying from it. The number of new AIDS cases in the United States went down in 1996 from 60,620 the year before to 56,730. That may not sound like a lot, but the 6 percent dip was the first-ever decline in the nearly 20-year history of this epidemic. While this is encouraging, it is still too early to tell if we have really turned the corner.

There was also a massive 23 percent decline in deaths from 1995 (when 50,700 people died of AIDS) to 1996 (39,200 deaths). Still, AIDS remains one of the leading causes of death among Americans between ages 25 and 44.

Winning the War

So what's going on here?

Well, three things, really. First of all, the number of Americans infected with the virus that causes AIDS—the human immunodeficiency virus, or HIV—seems to be dropping.

Formally (and somewhat arbitrarily) speaking, HIV infection is not acquired immunodeficiency syndrome, or AIDS. "After someone is infected with HIV, the virus and the immune system battle it out and there's a stalemate for a long time," says William Kassler, M.D., a medical epidemiologist with the Centers for Disease Control and Prevention and the chief of its health services, research, and evaluation branch in the division of STD (sexually transmitted disease) prevention, in Atlanta. "But eventually, the immune system tires out and the virus wins. And AIDS occurs when the immune system tires out."

And that's part two of what's going on. Therapies that didn't exist just a few years ago are now prolonging the stalemate.

"We now have drugs that come to the aid of the immune system and give it a chance to do its thing," Dr. Kassler says. "We have strategies to get the virus level in the bloodstream down to undetectable levels, though not zero."

And the third thing: Not only are new treatments delaying the progress of HIV to AIDS but also they're delaying the progress of AIDS to death.

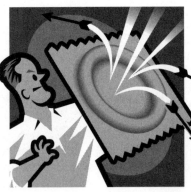

The thing about the HIV virus is that it mutates quickly. Just like crop pests, it builds up a resistance to whatever you're trying to zap it with. So the new successful treatments consist of complex and ever-shifting triple combinations of medications—the three-drug cocktails you may have heard about.

In actuality, there are something like 11 AIDS-fighting

drugs to choose from. All go after enzymes that help HIV replicate, either the reverse transcriptase enzyme or the protease enzyme.

"Once you burn up the drug, though—that is, once the virus gets resistant to it—you have to shuffle the deck and try another combination," Dr. Kassler says. "That's the challenge."

Then there's the biggest question mark. Will AIDS sufferers run out of different drugs to try before they run out of mutating viruses? "We haven't had these drugs around long enough to know," Dr. Kassler says. "And we don't know when the drugs are going to play themselves out."

The dream for AIDS, of course, is to find a cure, like penicillin was for syphilis. The hope for AIDS is to develop a vaccine, like for polio. But the current goal for AIDS, according to Dr. Kassler, is to turn it into a completely manageable disease, like diabetes.

Keeping HIV Away

AIDS may not yet be completely manageable, but it's completely preventable. And there's still plenty of incentive to prevent it.

For example, even while incidence in the United States is decreasing, worldwide rates of AIDS infection are soaring. While the rates for homosexual men are dropping, they're still high. And while the rates for heterosexual men are still low, they're rising. Any way you look at it, there's a problem out there.

Solve it by doing the right things. Let's assume that you, a health-minded individual, are not in the habit of shooting illegal drugs into your veins with used needles. There's part

How You Get It, How You Don't

According to Dr. William Kassler of the Centers for Disease Control and Prevention, you can get HIV from:

- *Sexual intercourse.* **With a woman or a man. Vaginal, anal, or oral. HIV can be in an infected person's blood, semen, or vaginal secretions and can enter the body through the moist lining of the penis, vagina, rectum, or mouth. It can also get in through sores, often so tiny that you don't even know you have them.**

- *Sharing needles.* **Even once. An infected person leaves HIV in a needle or syringe. An uninfected person shoots it right into his bloodstream.**

- *Getting a tattoo.* **Or your ears pierced. If the technician uses proper procedures and new or sterilized equipment, there's no danger. If it isn't done properly, there is.**

- *Getting blood products.* **It has happened in the past, most recently in other countries. But the screening procedures that the United States has adopted for its blood supply are so thorough that getting a transfusion is now considered extremely safe.**

On the other hand, Dr. Kassler says that you can't get HIV from:

- *Coughs or sneezes.* **HIV is not like a cold or flu virus. It doesn't fly through the air.**

- *Everyday contact.* **At school, work, home, or anywhere else.**

- *Giving blood.* **Due to the use of disposable equipment, this has never been a risk factor in the United States.**

- *Toilet seats.* **Or phones, clothes, forks, or cups.**

- *Mosquitoes.* **HIV isn't like the germ that causes malaria. It doesn't live in insects.**

- *Sweat, saliva, or tears.* **So kissing's safe, although it's possible that HIV can be transmitted through deep kissing because of potential, though unlikely, blood contact.**

of your AIDS risk taken care of. Virtually all the rest is from unprotected sexual relations. Protect your sex and you won't get AIDS, says Dr. Kassler.

Unprotected sex is dangerous because HIV can be transmitted through semen and vaginal secretions as well as blood. But if neither of you has HIV, then there's nothing to transmit. "If you're in a mutually monogamous relationship with somebody who is uninfected, that's safe sex," Dr. Kassler says. "You can do whatever you want."

That's simple enough, but it begs a question: How do you know? The sad fact is that you don't—unless you've both been recently tested or have been monogamous together long enough for any infections from previous relationships to declare themselves. Anybody can have HIV, and you can't tell just by looking at a person.

So protecting yourself against HIV and AIDS comes down to what you do and whom you do it with. "Limiting the number of people you have sex with helps," Dr. Kassler says. "However, choosing your partners wisely comes first." Here are a few other commonsense guidelines to follow.

Walk away from the wild side. Turn sex into a transaction and it turns dangerous. "That means that if you pay a prostitute or give out drugs in order to get sex, you're at increased risk for HIV," Dr. Kassler says. This isn't moral or legal advice; it's simply sound anti-AIDS strategy. "Those practices put you in contact with people who have the virus," Dr. Kassler says. "You're playing viral roulette."

Use your tongue. You've felt the tingle. Those few friendly dates reach critical mass and you just know that soon, tonight, in just a few hours, it's going to happen. You even

Lessons in Rubbership

Nobody ever said that using a condom comes naturally. How can you enjoy yourself if you're fighting the Trojan War? Here, courtesy of Dr. William Kassler of the Centers for Disease Control and Prevention, are the seven habits of highly effective and safe lovers.

Use latex. If you run across one of those old lambskin artifacts, don't use it for safe sex. It's porous enough for the virus to get through. Use latex or polyurethane condoms, which is what you'll almost always find in stores these days. Keep the lambskin version as a museum piece.

Stay current. That date on the package isn't the vintage. It's the last possible day you can safely use what's inside. Latex corrodes. So if your long-forgotten college stash of rubbers suddenly turns up, with a Cold War–era expiration date, put them in the same museum case as your lambskins.

Beat the heat. Heat will break down latex. That eliminates two favorite storage places for your condom supply—your wallet (body heat will do it) and anywhere in your car on warm days. Under the radiator or tucked in a lampshade are probably bad ideas as well.

Open with care. It's understood that sometimes the actual extraction of the condom from its packet is neces-

remembered to make the bed and cue up *Bolero* on the CD player. So what do you talk about at this critical turning point?

HIV, of course. What else?

The Centers for Disease Control actually did a study showing that discussing HIV with a new partner dramatically reduces the risk of contracting it. "Just asking a partner if they have been tested for HIV before you jump into bed is highly protective," Dr. Kassler says. "It works. You talk a little bit about it before you do it, and that's safer sex right there."

sarily performed in an atmosphere of, shall we say, urgency. But try to stay calm. If you start ripping at the wrapper with your fingernails or teeth or Swiss Army knife, you can inflict a surface wound on the condom itself that will defeat the purpose of using it. Take a deep breath, count to five, and gently tear. See how easy it can be?

Don't dawdle. Guys who thrust away and then don the condom just before ejaculating are, to put it generously, unclear on the concept. For one thing, your pre-ejaculate fluid can infect your partner if you're HIV-positive. And vaginal secretions can carry HIV to you. Put the condom on before there's any genital contact.

Roll with the flow. Condoms roll one way. So if you start to roll it the wrong way, you just turn it around and roll it the other way, right? Not if you want to protect your partner. You've already moistened what's now the outside of the condom, and the whole idea is to not exchange fluid. Throw it away and unroll another one.

Lube it right. Use water-based lubricants like K-Y Jelly or Astroglide. But don't use oil-based lubricants like Vaseline. They can break down the latex.

thing happened to me on the way to the clinic . . ."

Dr. Kassler suggests giving in order to get. "Volunteering information first may be the best way of getting the information from somebody else," he says. That would be the tell-all approach: "You're probably wondering this about me, so let me tell you that I . . ."

Use condoms . . . correctly and consistently. They've been the heroes of the epidemic and are as essential now as ever, especially with new partners. At some point, if you're in a long-term mutually monogamous relationship or you've both been tested, you can shed the latex. But in the meantime, use the condom from start to finish every time you have sex.

Take care of that little problem. Get yourself checked for other, less life-threatening STDs, and get them taken care of right away. Because herpes, syphilis, gonorrhea, or chlamydia puts you at increased risk for HIV. "It's not just that the person you got it from is more likely to have had HIV," Dr. Kassler says, "but also having an STD facilitates transmission of HIV. So if you have an STD and then get exposed to HIV, your risk of infection is 10 to 100 times greater."

If in doubt, get tested. Because your body produces telltale HIV antibodies when infected, a specific blood test for HIV can reveal whether you have it. The tests are sometimes free, sometimes anonymous, and always voluntary. While maintaining that the "latest medical knowledge gives added weight to the benefits of knowing if you are infected," the Centers for Disease Control's current opinion on testing is the following: "If you have engaged in behavior that can transmit HIV, it is very important that you consider counseling and testing."

A precoital HIV discussion may work, but it's not exactly an inherited courtship skill. Still, it's obviously worth it, so you're probably going to have to break the ice somehow. There's the apologetic approach: "Sorry I need to ask, but . . ." Or the we're-in-this-together approach: "Hey, you know, these days, times being what they are . . ." Or the suggestive approach: "Isn't this about the right time to talk about . . ." Or the non sequitur approach: "Speaking of HIV . . ." Or the tension-easing humorous approach: "A funny

Diabetes

Avoid Getting Type-Cast

Diabetes is the fourth leading cause of death in the United States, but very few people die directly from poorly controlled diabetes or diabetic coma these days. How's that? Consider this.

Diabetes itself is simply your body's inability to process the sugar, or glucose, in your bloodstream. There are two types. In type I (also known as immune-mediated diabetes or insulin-dependent diabetes), your pancreas stops producing insulin, the hormone you need to get the glucose into your cells. In type II, either your pancreas doesn't make enough insulin or your body doesn't use it right.

Type II is the one that you should really be concerned about, and it's the one we'll be telling you how to beat in this chapter. Type II's aliases are "adult-onset" or "non-insulin-dependent diabetes" or NIDDM (the *M* is for mellitus), and it's by far the most common—accounting for 9 out of 10 cases.

Fifteen million Americans have it. Eight million have it without knowing it.

But the most impressive fact is this: Most of adult-onset type II diabetes doesn't necessarily have to occur at all. "It's important to know that diabetes is preventable," says George King, M.D., associate professor of medicine at the Harvard Medical School and senior investigator of vascular cell biology at the Joslin Diabetes Center in Boston. "Or, if you have the disease, many complications can be prevented."

It's in Your Blood

If you were to die from acute complications of dia-betes such as a coma, you'd die from too much glucose in your bloodstream. And, sure enough, that's what used to happen before the discovery of insulin in 1922. But these days, diabetics can live happily and healthily ever after, by controlling their sugar intake to avoid complications. Those who have type I diabetes can also control their glucose levels with insulin shots, and those with type II can do so with a diet and exercise regimen, usually without insulin shots. Insufficiently controlled, however, either type of diabetes leads to other diseases—and that's where potentially fatal complications await.

The complications of diabetes read like a chamber of horrors. Heart attack, cardiovascular disease, stroke, and kidney failure are the most frequent causes of death. Diabetes also can lead to blindness, nerve disease, gangrene, lower limb amputation, and erectile dysfunction.

Somehow, a few minutes on a stationary bike and a strategic pass on the nachos doesn't seem like a lot to ask to avoid all that. Here are some other things you can do.

Just lose the weight. Low-fat? High-carbohydrate? Sprout-and-spinach-shake regimen? Don't worry about how you shed those extra pounds—at least as far as diabetes is concerned. Just shed them. "We don't really know if any specific diet works best for preventing type II diabetes," says Eli Ipp, M.D., head of the diabetes section at Harbor-UCLA Medical Center's division of endocrinology in Torrance, California. "The issue is to lose the weight and keep it off."

Exercise. Physical activity actually helps your body process glucose, so it helps prevent diabetic complications as well as the disease itself. In fact, medical researchers have actually taken disembodied human muscles, "exercised" them with electric stimulation, and then measured their insulin action. It works.

"Exercise can improve your insulin sensitivity a great deal no matter what your weight is," Dr. King says. "And the effects can last for two or three days."

Mix it up. Aerobic exercise is what's usually emphasized in the prevention of diabetes and its complications because that's what the subjects did in the studies that first made the connection. But new evidence shows that strength training and even offbeat activities such as tai chi can also improve insulin action, according to Aaron Vinik, M.D., Ph.D., director of research at the Diabetes Institute in Norfolk, Virginia. "All forms of activity have been shown to reduce the likelihood of complications once you have the disease," he says. "It doesn't have to be just aerobic exercise."

A caveat, though: Diabetics with nerve damage or eye disease should stay away from weight training because the strain of lifting weights can cause damaged blood vessels in the eyes to rupture and bleed, according to Dr. Vinik. And if you have nerve damage, you may not be able to sense the damage in your eyes.

Feel your oats. In a 1996 study, Canadian researchers fed four men bread made from oat bran for six months, while another four ate white bread. The oat bran–eaters showed better glucose levels. This finding is consistent with a 1997 study suggesting that diets that emphasize high-fiber whole grains (of which oat bran is one) over refined grains reduces your risk for type II diabetes.

Eliminate it with E. Free radicals— those pesky, tissue-damaging molecules—thrive on diabetes but succumb to antioxidants such as vitamin E.

Also, says Dr. King, vitamin E might help decrease complications for those with diabetes. "Since doses of 100 to 400 International Units are associated with a decrease in

---

Call Me, Sugar

Most people assume that sugar is virtually lethal for diabetics. Most people are wrong.

So were doctors for a century. The logic was that sugar = glucose = higher blood glucose levels. But it turns out that things don't work that way. Hence, the American Diabetes Association now acknowledges that table sugar as well as natural sugars such as fructose and lactose can be worked into a diabetic's meal plan.

Sugar alone may not directly raise your blood glucose level more than potatoes, for instance. But all its empty calories don't do anything for you but put on pounds. And the first order of business for beating diabetes is keeping your weight down.

---

heart disease, I would certainly take that much," he says.

Take your vitamin C. Vitamin C, another antioxidant plentiful in many fruits, may also do the trick. A 1995 study by an Italian research team linked vitamin C to improved glucose metabolism in type II diabetics.

Cool it with the booze. Teetotaling isn't required to fight diabetes, but anything more than one shot of liquor or one glass of wine or beer a day is asking for trouble, according to Dr. King. "If you drink too much, you can damage your pancreas," he warns. "And that's where the insulin comes from in the first place."

Watch for the warning signs. Forewarned is forearmed. According to the American Diabetes Association, the following are worth seeing a doctor about: increased thirst; increased need to urinate; an edgy, tired, and sick-to-the-stomach feeling; repeated or hard-to-heal infections of your skin, gums, or bladder; blurred vision; tingling or loss of feeling in your hands or feet; dry, itchy skin.

Other Diseases

Protection from Head to Toe

When the topic is mortality, heart disease and cancer get most of the attention. And for good reason: No other cause of death, including accidents, comes close to either of them.

But if heart disease and cancer alone account for slightly more than half of all deaths in the United States (which they do), that means that all the others account for only slightly *less* than half. Attacking anywhere from your brain to your bowel, the Grim Reaper's supporting cast can kill you just as dead as the Big Two. Or they can color the rest of your years varying shades of miserable.

Here, then, from top to bottom, are some more potential enemies and ways to keep them out of your life.

Trouble on the Brain

Any dementia-causing neurological condition can slowly rob you of things you take for granted—like language, memory, judgment, even your ability to make sense of what you see or where you are. Alzheimer's disease is the most common form of dementia and perhaps the deadliest. The estimated four million American adults who have it suffer any combination of those cognitive losses, usually starting off with seemingly insignificant memory lapses.

There are genes that predispose you to Alzheimer's. A family history of any kind of dementia puts you at higher risk. Other risk factors include a his-

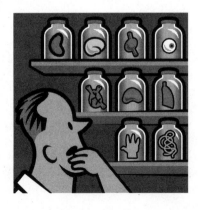

tory of depression, alcohol abuse, or thyroid disease. Here are some ways to bolster your odds against this ailment.

Get smart. An idle mind is Alzheimer's playground. "Well-educated people seem to show signs of Alzheimer's less often," says Linda Hershey, M.D., Ph.D., professor of neurology at the State University of New York at Buffalo and chief of neurology at the Veterans Affairs Medical Center, also in Buffalo. "Education has a protective effect."

But even if you dropped out of school, it's not too late to build up your brain against Alzheimer's. Dedication to mind-challenging hobbies like music, cards, or drawing will help, according to the Institute for Brain Aging and Dementia at the University of California, Irvine, College of Medicine. The only requirement is an active mind.

Relieve brain pain. A toxic protein in Alzheimer's patients' brains actually stimulates inflammatory reactions that contribute to cell loss. "You could possibly slow that process by taking an anti-inflammatory pain remedy like ibuprofen," Dr. Hershey says. "Just like this drug helps reduce inflammation in your joints, it helps the same way in your brain." In fact, studies have shown that any of the nonsteroid anti-inflammatory drugs (that is, aspirin, ibuprofen, and the like) help. But Dr. Hershey cautions that you should ask your physician before taking these drugs, as they can cause serious side effects.

Take vitamin E. When Columbia University researchers looked at Alzheimer's sufferers, they found that those who took vitamin E in the middle stages took about a year longer before requiring institutionalization. That doesn't mean that vitamin E can prevent Alzheimer's. Also, this study's dosage was much higher than what most doctors would recommend. In fact, taking high doses of vitamin E has the potential to cause neuropathy, according to Dr. Hershey.

"Vitamin E presumably works because it's an antioxidant and, therefore, the enemy of free radicals that can damage brain cells in people with Alzheimer's," Dr. Hershey says. "A free-radical scavenger like vitamin E can slow down the process." And so can other antioxidants, research indicates, including ginkgo and vitamin C. But again, before you add a vitamin E supplement to your diet, Dr. Hershey advises that you speak with your doctor.

Watch your head. Trauma, especially combined with a predisposing gene, increases your risk for Alzheimer's. It can happen from one severe head injury, or various blows to the noggin over the years. "If you have the gene, head trauma can make the symptoms show up earlier," Dr. Hershey says.

Check the pressure. High blood pressure is usually associated with other kinds of dementia, but at least one study at the University of Illinois has found a hypertension-Alzheimer's link. Fifteen years after having their blood pressure tracked at age 70, those in the study group who developed Alzheimer's turned out to be those with higher blood pressure readings.

Tales of the Lung

Breathing's pretty much what it's all about in the death-defying game. But more than 96,000 Americans each year stop doing it thanks to an increasingly rampant form of lung disease called chronic obstructive pulmonary disease, or COPD. This isn't

Eye on Glaucoma

At least two million Americans have glaucoma, the second leading cause of preventable vision loss after diabetes. The disease—a result of extra pressure on the optic nerve from improperly draining eye fluid—isn't curable, but it's treatable, often with pressure-reducing eyedrops.

In other words, you don't have to go blind if you get glaucoma. But some people do.

"There's no excuse for vision loss from glaucoma other than personal neglect," insists Richard Bensinger, M.D., a spokesman for the American Academy of Ophthalmologists in Seattle. "Either you never got your eyes checked or your physician didn't nag you hard enough to follow the medical regimen."

Why should you have to be nagged into not going blind? According to Dr. Bensinger, it's not just the mild inconvenience of an eyedrop routine but also the lack of immediate payoff. "We don't have to encourage people with arthritis because they're hurting, and when they take their medicine, the pain goes away," he says. "But with glaucoma the results seem like nothing. You don't see any better or feel any better after you take the drops."

There's a similar reluctance about eye checkups, even though if you catch glaucoma in the bud via an eye-pressure test, you keep most of your sight. "The problem is that garden-variety glaucoma doesn't have any symptoms," Dr. Bensinger says.

So don't wait till it's too late. Dr. Bensinger recommends that you get your eyes examined every five years from age 25 to 50, and every two years after that. And you should have your eyes checked more often if there is a history of glaucoma in your family.

And please, take your medicine.

pneumonia or lung cancer but a group of conditions characterized by blocked air flow.

There are two principal players in this death act—chronic bronchitis and emphysema—and they often do a duet in the same victim. You may have had a bout with acute bronchitis, with all that coughing and mucus accompanying a severe cold. Imagine those symptoms as a permanent result of inflamed and scarred bronchial tubes and you know what chronic bronchitis is all about.

Emphysema weakens and breaks the inner walls of the air sacs in the lungs, impairing the flow of air into the lungs and the distribution of oxygen into the rest of the body. The damage is irreversible, and emphysema victims find themselves short of breath and unable to do much of anything that requires physical exertion.

About 14 million Americans suffer from chronic bronchitis (a 60 percent increase since 1982), and 2 million from emphysema, 61 percent of them male. The cause of this sad state of affairs is smoking, for the most part. It accounts for 82 percent of all COPD. Don't smoke, and you're 82 percent of the way there. Here are some other ways to keep on breathing.

Find clean air. Hawaii might start looking pretty good to you if you're in the early stages of COPD. The best way to control chronic bronchitis is to keep your nose, throat, sinuses, and bronchial tubes away from things that can inflame or irritate them, says Dr. Steven Mostow of the University of Colorado. Those things include smog, dusty working conditions, and cigarette smoke. Air pollution also aggravates emphysema symptoms. If Hawaii's out of the question, the American Lung Association recommends that you plan your activities in the early morning or evening when smog levels are at their lowest.

Skirting STDs

It seems like when AIDS came on the scene in the early 1980s we pretty much forgot about all the other sexually transmitted diseases (STDs). But they didn't forget about us. STDs are a hidden epidemic, newly infecting 12 million Americans a year. They haven't gone away.

Here's a roster of the heavy hitters.

Herpes simplex 2. This version of herpes may have found a home by now in as many as one in four sexually active men, two-thirds of whom don't know they have it. When the characteristic open sores show themselves in the genital area, that's when you can usually catch it—or give it. "But you can also actually pass it on to a sex partner when a lesion is nowhere in sight," says Dr. William Kassler of the Centers for Disease Control and Prevention. "That's what has everybody concerned. We think it's what's fueling the herpes epidemic."

Chlamydia. It's the fastest-spreading STD, infecting as many as four million men and women a year. It's a particularly insidious one, too, since men don't have symptoms about a quarter of the time, and women three-quarters of the time. When symptoms do show up, you'll probably experience either a genital discharge, painful urination, or both. Chlamydia also, though rarely, can cause painful or swollen testicles. Chlamydia is a bacterial infection, so it's curable with antibiotics—if you know that you have it.

Genital warts. Its given name is human papillomavirus, or HPV. The symptoms are what its nickname implies—warts on the anus, penis, or scrotum. About a million Americans join the HPV club each year. They never leave it.

Syphilis. This one has been rockin' longer than Mick and Keith. It's one of the more manageable STDs these days since it usually makes its presence known via a painless chancre on the penis and exits promptly with antibiotics. Ignore it, however, and it can result in blindness, heart disease, and death.

Gonorrhea. The symptoms are similar to those of chlamydia. Also like chlamydia, the symptoms sometimes fail to show up. The clap gets about 800,000 Americans each year but succumbs nicely to antibiotics.

Hepatitis B. Like HIV, it's found in blood, semen, and vaginal secretions and is spread through sexual contact and shared needles. Unlike HIV, it usually clears itself up in a month or two. But this kind of hepatitis needs medical attention because possible liver damage puts you at risk for cirrhosis or liver cancer.

You can keep from getting any of these STDs by following much the same safe-sex guidelines that you do for AIDS—careful partner selection, mutual full disclosure before sex, and a strict adherence to condom use, says Dr. Kassler.

And for most STDs, you have an option you don't have with AIDS—getting rid of it. "The thing to do is recognize the symptoms of STDs, go to a doctor, and get them treated," Dr. Kassler says. "The earlier you get them taken care of, the safer you are."

Nip infections early. Any cold or respiratory infection is going to make COPD symptoms worse. So it's not wimpy to consult a doctor at the first sniffle of a cold. And ask your doctor about getting vaccinated against influenza and pneumococcal pneumonia, two illnesses that can severely hinder breathing, says Dr. Mostow.

Keep moving. COPD or no, general health is still a good way to fight off infections. The American Lung Association recommends regular exercise that doesn't tire you out much for chronic bronchitis sufferers. You should also exercise with emphysema, but as part of a doctor-guided pulmonary rehabilitation program, says Dr. Mostow.

Beating Asthma

Asthma gets separate billing from COPD in the rogue's gallery. But it's also a lung disease. It's also chronic. It's also life-threatening. And about five million American men have it in one form or another.

Asthmatics have hyperactive bronchial tubes in the lungs that can be triggered into breath-robbing spasms by allergic reactions to things such as animal dander, mold spores, or pollen, or by environmental irritants such as smog, cold air, or tobacco smoke.

It doesn't go away. If you have asthma, you live with it. But there are ways to make living with it a lot easier.

Pull the triggers. Asthma attacks don't just happen. Something triggers them, and those triggers vary with the victim. They can be anything from dust to gases to allergies to viruses. The best way to get control over asthma, according to the American Lung Association, is to discover what conditions set off the attacks. Then avoid those conditions.

Stay out of the ozone.
Ozone takes a particularly heavy toll on asthmatics, according to Dr. Bill McDonnell of the U.S. Environmental Protection Agency. "Asthma tends to be worse for several days following high-ozone days," Dr. McDonnell says. "That might be manifested in more symptoms of asthma, more medication use, or more trips to emergency rooms." But you may be able to avoid trips to the emergency room by limiting periods of outdoor exercise to times when ozone concentrations are low in your area, typically early mornings, adds Dr. McDonnell.

Take a dip. Exercise can sometimes trigger asthma attacks, but you can still exercise if you have asthma. Swimming might be the best way to do it because breathing warm, moist air at a pool is better for your airways than cool, dry air, says Dr. Mostow. Or you can try warming the air you breathe by wearing a scarf over your nose and mouth as you exercise. A longer warmup—at least 15 minutes—might also help.

Milk magnesium. Long known for its ability to relax the muscles lining our breathing passages, research shows that magnesium may even help fend off an asthma attack, says Richard J. Wood, Ph.D., associate professor at the School of Nutrition at Tufts University in Medford, Massachusetts, and laboratory chief of the Mineral Bioavailability Laboratory. Get your magnesium from seeds, beans, nuts, and dark green vegetables such as spinach and Swiss chard.

Have a cup of coffee. The caffeine molecule is a lot like the molecules of the compound in the sprays that asthmatics use to relax the bronchial spasms. A cup of joe isn't as effective as a bronchodilator, of course, but it goes a lot better with the morning newspaper.

Travel Safe

Mountain climbing in Nepal. Scuba diving in Honduras. Gorilla watching in Rwanda. If you don't travel, you're reading only one page in the book of life.

But if you do travel, you're at risk for diseases virtually unheard of in the good old United States. "Of the 20 million Americans who leave the country each year, 2 million to 3 million go into what we call the Third World," says Dr. Steven Mostow of the University of Colorado. "And the incidence of disease is very high in that group of countries."

Examples include cholera, malaria, and dengue fever. Tuberculosis, too, is on the rise worldwide (in the United States, too, in this case). And remember, while AIDS seems to have stabilized in the United States, cases are soaring worldwide. Plus, in some places—Africa, for example—it's much more prevalent among heterosexuals, so the high-risk sexual preferences are flip-flopped.

Even what seems like child's play here is deadly in some parts of the world. "In some Third World environments, measles is still a wild, uncontrolled disease," Dr. Mostow says. "And chickenpox is probably the most contagious virus in the world."

Arthritis Strategies

This piece of information may not make your day, but there are more than 100 kinds of arthritis inflicting their brand of pain on the

Furthermore, Dr. Mostow points out, a lot of adventurous travelers aren't exactly a $3 cab fare away from first-rate treatment. "Papua New Guinea, for example, has some of the best diving in the world," he says. "But if you contract measles there, you're in deep doo-doo. The medical care is as primitive as the rest of the island."

There's a name for all this: emporiatrics, the study of the diseases of the emerging world. And there's a way to deal with it as well: travel medicine clinics that specialize in getting you there and back disease-free.

"If you visit a travel clinic before you travel, your chances of getting ill are greatly reduced," says Dr. Mostow, who set up one such clinic, Rose Travel Medicine, in Denver. "You get all the right shots and information on the food-borne diseases and sexually transmitted diseases. We also go through how you deal with a consulate if you're in trouble and give you a list of competent doctors who speak English."

Remember, those visa-required shots are to protect the country you're going to from *you*, not the other way around. That's one reason that travel clinics make sense if your itinerary includes places more exotic than the grand tour of Europe.

Doctors treat arthritis with anti-inflammatory drugs and physical therapy. But you can do some things on your own to reduce the need for their services.

Ease the burden. Research shows what common sense dictates: Your joints do better if you put less weight on them. "On average, population surveys indicate that for every 10 pounds you lose, you decrease the occurrence of arthritis by 50 percent," says David Pisetsky, M.D., Ph.D., professor of medicine and chief of research at the Duke University Arthritis Center in Durham, North Carolina. "If you're overweight, get back as close to your normal body weight as you can."

Don't be too smashing. Play rough and you push up your risk for arthritis. "If you play football, to use an extreme example, you're subject to joint injury all the time," Dr. Pisetsky says. "That increases the likelihood of arthritis." But that doesn't mean that you should go motionless. "Exercise is likely to decrease the symptoms of arthritis," Dr. Pisetsky says. Make that moderate exercise. Go easy on those extreme sports.

Take your vitamins. Research indicates that vitamin B_{12} stimulates bone-generating osteoblasts, which could stem the forward march of arthritis. Vitamins E and C have also received some support for pain relief and cartilage repair because of their antioxidant qualities. "We know that oxidative damage occurs in the joints, and studies have indicated that people who have increased their intake of antioxidants may have less arthritis," Dr. Pisetsky says. "There's a lot of interest in it, but it's not at a point yet where we can make definite recommendations." In the meantime, Dr. Pisetsky recommends packing

joints of some 17 million American men (and 23 million women).

In osteoarthritis (the most common), the underlying bone of a joint degenerates because the protective cartilage has broken down over time. Rheumatoid arthritis, on the other hand, can affect younger people because the inflammation is the result not of wear and tear but of the body's own immune cells doing a Benedict Arnold act on the joints.

your diet full of antioxidant-rich foods and for older men to take add a multivitamin to their diets.

Up your fish ante. The oils in fish contain the friendly polyunsaturated fats called omega-3 fatty acids. Scientists can measure a significant drop in inflammatory immune substances if there's enough fish oil in your diet. That means less morning stiffness and tender joints if you have rheumatoid arthritis. Fish with the most omega-3 to offer include herring, salmon, mackerel, and tuna.

Rout the gout. Gout is one form of arthritis more common in men than women. You get it from too much uric acid, so cut down on anything that creates uric acid, says Dr. Pisetsky. That includes alcohol, and purine-rich foods such as anchovies, mussels, fish roe, and organ meat.

Disease Down Under

A young man, they say, will do anything for sex. A middle-age man will do anything for money. An older man will do anything for respect. But all men will do anything for a good bowel movement.

The problem is that a lot can go wrong between digestion and elimination, irritable bowel syndrome being an all-too-common example. IBS, as it's affectionately called, isn't life-threatening and doesn't lead to harder stuff like colorectal cancer. It isn't inflammatory and doesn't permanently damage the bowel. In fact, it's not really a disease but, rather, a "functional disorder."

The function it disorders is bowel movement. You can have painful constipation with difficult or infrequent bowel movements. Or you can have equally painful diarrhea with a lot of loose stools and urgent desires to reduce the real estate between your irritable bowel and a toilet. Or you can enjoy both versions. Adding to the pleasure are crampy abdominal pain, gassiness, and bloating.

As bad as IBS sounds (and feels), it's not nearly as serious as inflammatory bowel disease, or IBD. This is a group of disorders that cause inflammation and ulceration in the small and large intestines. Ulcerative colitis and Crohn's disease, the two major members of the IBD family, cause symptoms similar to IBS. But they also can offer nasty bonuses—like rectal bleeding, weight loss, fever, anemia.

Doctors aren't sure what causes IBS or IBD. They do know that unlike IBS, IBD has a genetic element to it; 20 percent of people with Crohn's disease have a blood relative with some form of inflammatory bowel disease. There's no cure for either one, though treatment under a doctor's care can ease the discomfort. So can the following recommendations from the National Institutes of Health.

Assess your food. Milk products, large amounts of alcohol, avocados, and excess fat of any kind can contract your bowel in inconvenient ways. But different folks react to different foods, so the National Institutes of Health recommends that you actually keep a journal of the relationship between what goes in and how it comes out. It's not exactly the kind of diary material that made Samuel Pepys famous, but it could help you avoid undue distress from IBS.

Don't overeat. Those seven-course extravaganzas can cause cramping and diarrhea in people with IBS. Try smaller meals more often or just eat smaller portions. And keep the fiber high and the fat low. High-fiber diets mildly distend the colon (the largest section of the bowel, or large intestine), and that helps prevent symptom-starting spasms from developing. You may feel some bloating when you first up the fiber, but that should stop as your body adjusts to the better diet.

Lessen your stress. Another trigger for IBS symptoms is emotional stress, which can also aggravate the symptoms of IBD simply by increasing the number of bowel movements.

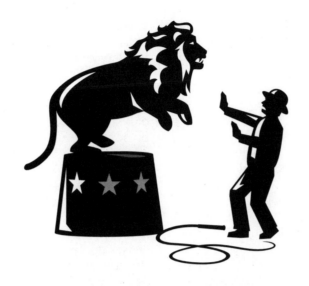

Part Four

Beating the Men-Killers

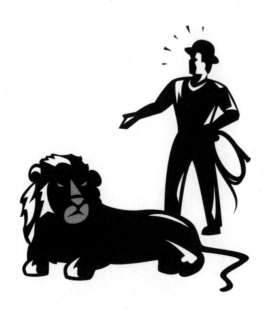

The Accidental Dead Guy

Bumping Into Your Maker

In the 10 minutes it takes to read this chapter, 2 people will be killed and 370 will be disabled by an unintentional injury. By the time an hour goes by, 11 people will die an "accidental" death, and an astonishing 2,200 will be disabled by an accident. And guess what? Most of them will be men.

Fortunately, we're finally beginning to get smarter about safety, says Jeffrey Sacks, M.D., medical epidemiologist at the National Center for Injury Prevention and Control, division of unintentional injury prevention, at the Centers for Disease Control and Prevention in Atlanta. "There has been a proliferation of safety devices in our lives," Dr. Sacks says. "But honestly, we can still be pretty dumb about using them. And way, way too often, alcohol and drugs are a factor in our lack of judgment."

Different Endings

It'll be of little surprise to anyone that one place we exercise the worst judgment and pay for it the most is on the road, where more fatal accidents happen than anywhere else. But we also do quite a number on ourselves at the workplace and—even worse—in our own homes. Here are the top types of fatal accidents and steps that safety experts say you can take to avoid bumping into your maker before your time.

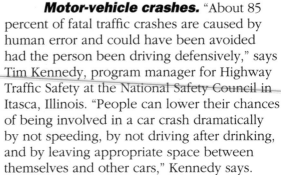

Motor-vehicle crashes. "About 85 percent of fatal traffic crashes are caused by human error and could have been avoided had the person been driving defensively," says Tim Kennedy, program manager for Highway Traffic Safety at the National Safety Council in Itasca, Illinois. "People can lower their chances of being involved in a car crash dramatically by not speeding, by not driving after drinking, and by leaving appropriate space between themselves and other cars," Kennedy says.

Falls. Each year more than a million folks get a trip to the hospital for a trip down the stairs. Aside from exercising caution, experts say that regular exercise—especially exercises that emphasize balance, such as tai chi—can help you maintain your coordination and stay on your feet throughout your life.

Poisonings I—solids and liquids. We tend to think of poisoning as something that happens when little kids get into medicine cabinets, but people ages 25 to 44 are actually six feet under everyone else when it come to this brand of accidental death—with twice the death rate of toddlers. If you suspect that you or someone else has "overdosed" on drugs or medication or has swallowed something poisonous, call your local poison control center. More than 70 percent of poisonings can be treated through instructions taken over the phone, says Alton Thygerson, Ed.D., professor of health science at Brigham Young University in Provo, Utah, and technical consultant to the National Safety Council's First-Aid Institute in Itasca, Illinois.

Drowning. About 85 percent of all drowning victims are men, says Dr. Thygerson. Drowning kills about 4,500 people a year. When the victims are adult men, alcohol is a factor most of the time, Dr. Thygerson says. "We can't seem to get it through to people that drinking and boating and swimming are deadly combinations. Save it for the shore."

Fires. About 4,700 people die each year because of fires—the majority of which are avoidable, says Susan McKelvey, public affairs manager of the National Fire Protection Association in Quincy, Massachusetts. "Taking basic safety precautions greatly reduces the risk of fire," McKelvey says. "Cigarettes should be extinguished with water; smoking carelessly is the leading cause of fire death in the United States. Don't leave the kitchen when you're cooking; cooking is the leading cause of fires. And it's recommended that you have at least one smoke detector on every level of your home as well as in or near all sleeping areas," she says. Simple steps like these can significantly improve your safety from fire.

Choking. About 1,500 people every year die when they accidentally inhale a bit of food or a foreign object and it becomes lodged in their windpipes. Dr. Thygerson recommends that everyone know how to perform abdominal thrusts (the Heimlich maneuver). For a conscious victim, wrap your arms around the victim's waist from behind. Make a fist with one hand, and place the thumb side just above the victim's navel. Grasp that fist with your other hand and press it up and into the victim's abdomen until whatever is blocking the airway is expelled. You can perform this on yourself, says Dr. Thygerson, by pressing the abdomen (slightly above the navel) quickly over any firm surface, such as the back of a chair, side of a table, or porch railing.

For complete instructions on rescuing a choking victim, or getting cardiopulmonary resuscitation (CPR) certification, contact your local American Red Cross or American Heart Association.

Firearms. Unintentional shootings claim

Darwin Had a Point

Scientist Charles Darwin championed a concept known as survival of the fittest. In the spirit of this great scientist, there is a group of folks on the Internet bestowing what's known as the Darwin Awards on humans who have effectively removed themselves from the gene pool in the stupidest of ways.

You bet your life. A 26-year-old man was killed in Selbyville, Delaware, after acting on a bet with friends who said he would not put a loaded revolver into his mouth and pull the trigger. At least he won the bet.

Look before you leap. Another 26-year-old man in Mulberry, Indiana, broke his neck after diving into one foot of water at a local marina.

Watch that high tide. A 21-year-old Colorado man got out of a truck's cab and acted like he was "surfing the waves" in the back. The driver took a turn and threw him out of the bed. The surfer was pronounced dead at the scene.

about 1,500 lives each year. And men are almost six times more likely to die at the smoky end of a misfired gun than women. If you have a gun at home, be sure that you and everyone in the house know firearm safety. Keep bullets and guns safely locked away, preferably in different places, says Michael Taylor, manager of the community safety division at the National Safety Council.

Poisonings II—gases and vapors. If you don't have a carbon monoxide detector on each level of your house, you should, says Taylor. Four hundred people each year die from being exposed to poisonous gases and vapors, in particular, carbon monoxide. Cooking and heating equipment as well as idling motor vehicles are major sources of this colorless, odorless, lethal gas.

Auto Accidents

Driving Us to Our Grave

Way back in 1769, Nicholas Joseph Cugnot took his newly invented, self-propelled, steam-driven automobile prototype out for its maiden voyage. Humming around his Parisian neighborhood at about 2½ miles per hour, Cugnot whacked into a wall, knocking it down, thereby putting the very first automobile accident on the books.

Just look what he started. Every year about 10.7 million auto accidents are added to the roster. From those accidents, about 2.3 million people end up with disabling injuries. And 44,000 end up dead. It's statistics like these that make the venerated road trip one of the most dangerous activities that everyday folks do. More people die in cars for every 100 million miles traveled than they do in planes, trains, or buses.

"Car crashes are the leading cause of death for people ages 1 to 34," says Stephanie Faul, communications director of the American Automobile Association's (AAA) Foundation for Traffic Safety in Washington, D.C. "Driving is the most dangerous thing the average person does every day." That said, driving isn't nearly as deadly as it used to be, thanks to public education about safety and better engineering in the automobile industry. But we still have a long way to go, says Faul.

A Safer Ride

Most of us can remember a day not too long ago when the biggest safety feature in cars were lap belts that nobody bothered wearing. Then came shoulder belts. Soon after, safety bugs and crash test dummies were ap-

pearing in public service announcements telling us that buckling up saves lives. States started making it illegal not to wear a seat belt. Today, cars are sold as much by their plethora of safety features like antilock brakes and daytime running lights as they are by cost and color.

The safety push has paid off. During the past 80 years, the number of deaths for every 10,000 registered passenger vehicles has plummeted 94 percent. Way back in 1912, there were 3,100 car crash deaths on record, even though there were only 950,000 registered vehicles driving on U.S. roads. In 1995, almost 44,000 people died on American roadways, but we also had more than 204 million registered cars driving around out there. Just wearing seat belts has saved almost 10,000 lives during the past 10 years, say statisticians.

"If folks were willing, we could make cars even safer," says Tim Kennedy of the National Safety Council, pointing to the National Association of Stock Car Racing (NASCAR) drivers who routinely emerge from their mangled wreckage unscathed. "If we were willing to wear helmets and five-point safety belts that crossed both shoulders and around our waists, we could be a whole lot safer. We could also build cages inside our cars like Indy drivers have. But there's only so much the public is willing to accept."

The Great Air Bag Debate

One of the most successful car safety inventions in recent years doesn't require you to do anything—one of the reasons, perhaps, for its success. We're talking about the air bag. When it comes to head-on collisions, air bags help reduce the death rate by about 34 percent. While it's true that in certain circumstances an inflating air bag can actually cause injury, those cases are generally avoidable and also pale in comparison to the number of lives that air bags have saved. The key to getting the full-blown benefits from your air bags is proper usage. Here's how.

Buckle everyone in. "Unfortunately, many, if not most, of the people who have been hurt by inflating air bags were not properly restrained," Kennedy says. "Never rely on the air bag alone to save you. You and your passengers, in the front and back, should always wear your seat belts. Younger children—up to 6 years old—according to their size and your state's regulation, should always be in approved child safety seats." When taking Junior to batting practice, be sure he's securely buckled up in the back seat if he's younger than 12. The impact of an inflating air bag can be fatally overpowering for kids. The same is true for infants in child seats. Always keep them in the back, properly restrained, adds Kennedy.

Use the 10-inch rule. The Department of Transportation recommends that people sit as far away from the steering wheel as possible, while still having full control of the car. If you can hold a piece of paper lengthwise—roughly 10 inches—between your chest and the steering wheel hub, that's a safe distance.

Move up, not in. Not everyone is 5 feet 10 inches or taller. And not everyone can comfortably see over the dashboards of bigger cars and trucks. If you're one of them, don't squeeze in close to the dash to peer over. Kennedy's suggestion: Buy a "booster cushion," which lifts you a couple of inches, instead. If you're dreading getting ragged by your buddies, buy one for the passenger seat, too, then cover both with seat covers. You'll both see better on your next trip and be safer, too.

Car Talk

There's no doubt that your cellular phone can get you out of a big bind when that 10-minute jaunt to an important meeting across town becomes a 45-minute traffic snarl. But hang on the line longer than to say, "Hey, I'm running late," and you may be running into trouble.

Canadian researchers studied almost 700 people with cellular phones in their cars who had been in an accident. They found that the risk for having an accident while gabbing on your cell phone increased four times— a risk rate similar to the risk of drinking and driving. And it didn't matter if their hands were tied up with a handheld phone or if they kept their mitts free by using a hands-free model; the risk was the same. That said, research shows that dumping your cell phone isn't the answer either since they're mighty important in emergency situations. Out of the study volunteers who had a cell phone–related accident, 39 percent then used their car phone to call for help.

Drive Yourself Sober

If you're thinking of driving after drinking, think first of this sobering fact: More than 40 percent of fatal crashes involve a driver or pedestrian who had been drinking. "It doesn't make any sense to gamble and hope that you're not the one affected. Don't be so cocky to ignore the risks," says Kennedy. You're also forcing everyone who crosses your path to take the same risk. Nearly half of the people killed in crashes are innocent victims killed by drivers who had a few—or less than a few.

So try heeding the following advice from safety experts to help reduce your risk of being involved in an alcohol-related accident.

Use common sense. Some people stick to the guideline of having one drink an hour, followed by a nonalcoholic drink in the second hour, to monitor their blood alcohol level, says James Fell, chief of research and evaluation at the National Highway Traffic Safety Administration in Washington, D.C. "But we really can't say what a safe BAC is because everyone is affected differently, considering their age, weight, fat, food intake, and experience. The motto, plain and simple," Fell adds, "is that if you have to drive, don't drink. If you have to drink, don't drive."

Act like it's New Year's Eve. People have a heightened awareness of how dangerous the roads and highways are when everyone's out ringing in the New Year, says Kennedy. "Well, any time you're on the road late at night, especially on the weekends, you are driving among a lot of people who have been drinking," he says.

Be aware of your surroundings. Keep yourself safe by leaving plenty of room between you and the cars around you. And by all means, don't challenge anyone's reaction time by making a quick turn in front of another car or cutting into traffic, Kennedy says. "Just being mindfully aware of the potential danger can keep you safer," he advises.

A Need to Heed Speed

When engineers make roads, they take a lot of factors into consideration before telling you how fast you can go, Kennedy says. "Those numbers you see indicating the speed limit aren't arbitrary. Road engineers consider the population of the neighborhood, the angle of the curves, the volume of traffic, and numerous other factors to figure the maximum speed you can safely travel," he says.

The problem is that lots of folks choose to ignore the limits. Going faster than the posted speed limit contributes to more than 68 percent of fatal car crashes, according to the National Safety Council.

You don't have to have your foot through the floorboards to get killed in a speed-related crash either. Only about 13 percent of speeding-related deaths occur on high-speed interstate highways. The rest happen as folks are flying around their familiar stomping grounds, generally after they've been drinking.

The take-home message here is to slow the heck down. You risk killing not just yourself but also some innocent mom, dad, or child who crosses your path, says Kennedy.

It's All the Rage

You know that jackass who insists on driving about 10 miles per hour below the speed limit? The one who inspires Walter Mitty fantasies of you piloting a monster truck, crushing his little Volkswagen like the bug it is? Well, while Sunday drivers have always been a little frustrating, these days they're downright deadly because increasingly, people are moving from mumbling and gesticulating at bad drivers to ramming them with their cars and, occasionally, shooting them.

This phenomenon has become so common that it even has a name: road rage. And it's getting worse. According to AAA data, the incidence of drivers outwardly expressing their hostility at one another for actions committed on the road—the formal definition of road rage—has been increasing by about 7 percent each year since 1990.

Short of taking the train, what's a poor driving stiff to do, especially when you feel your blood boil when some jerk bobs and weaves around you on your morning commute? Here's what Arnold P. Nerenberg, Ph.D., a clinical psychologist in private practice in Whittier, California, suggests.

Consider the consequences. Before you start your engine, think how much it could cost you financially as well as physically to get all wound up on your trip, suggests Dr. Nerenberg. "Recognize that your problem of acting hostile to other drivers could cost you your life if an accident occurs or someone shoots you," he says. "You could be sued for causing an accident, not to mention the toll it takes on your health to get all upset."

Get a head start. If road rage is a problem for you, always leave 15 minutes earlier for your destination than you think you should, Dr. Nerenberg says. "That way you won't be irritated from the get-go because you're in a hurry," he says.

Night Terrors

Aggressive and drunken driving are far from the sole contributors to auto accidents and fatalities. Statistics show that many factors—some you'd never consider, like drowsiness or even the way you drive at night—contribute to death on the roadways as well. Here's what you need to know to cover all your safety bases on the road.

Sleep on it. Driving without sleep can be as dangerous as driving after drinking. And the effects of sleep deprivation are so pronounced that researchers found that there is an increase in the number of auto accidents on the Monday after daylight saving time begins (when we lose an hour of sleep) and a decrease in accidents the Monday after the fall change back (when we gain an hour). "Take your sleep seriously," says Faul.

Spit shine those high beams. "Accidents often occur at night because of poor visibility," says Kennedy. One surefire solution is to

---

The Best of Drives, The Worst of Drives

Fort Lauderdale, Florida, may have been a kickin' place to do Spring Break back in your Lambda Chi days. But as the city with the highest auto-accident fatality rate in the nation—25.18 for every 100,000 people—it's not the place to be if you want to stay safe on the road. Here are the three best and the three worst cities and states for auto accidents, according to the Bureau of Census.

City	Auto Deaths per 100,000
Best	
1. Worcester, Massachusetts	3.02
2. Irving, Texas	3.03
3. Providence, Rhode Island	3.98
Worst	
1. Fort Lauderdale, Florida	25.18
2. Tampa, Florida	24.52
3. Salt Lake City, Utah	20.95

State	Death Rate per 100 Million Miles Traveled
Best	
1. Massachusetts/Rhode Island (tie)	0.9
2. Connecticut/New Hampshire (tie)	1.1
3. New Jersey/Vermont (tie)	1.3
Worst	
1. Mississippi	2.8
2. Arkansas	2.4
3. Nevada/Louisiana (tie)	2.3

---

slow it down an extra notch in the nighttime to give yourself extra stopping and steering time, he says. Another may be to clean those headlights of yours. Dirt on your car's headlights can lessen their light output by 75 percent.

Accidents in the Home

The Handyman's Downfall

Everyone wants to be like Bob Vila, the ultimate safe, competent handyman. But in reality, most of us are more like *Home Improvement*'s Tim "The Toolman" Taylor, an accident waiting to happen.

More often than not, our attempts at home improvement don't mean more trips to the local hardware superstore, but to the emergency room instead, says Michael Taylor (no relation to Tim "The Toolman") of the National Safety Council, who specializes in home safety awareness. "Not that we try to discourage people from working on things around the house. But they should know their limits. And they should know what they're doing," he says. "People have this misconception that they are magically safe within their own homes, when, in fact, that's where most accidents happen."

Fall from Grace

If we could prevent falls, we could prevent hundreds of thousands of disabling injuries and deaths in the home. Here are some tips for staying on your feet, as well as guidelines if you find yourself unexpectedly swept off them.

Watch that last step. Need we say it? The instant you feel you're putting yourself in danger for a fall, you are, Taylor says. "Move the ladder; don't reach from the top rungs. Don't reach for something from the

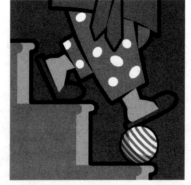

edge of the roof. Use stepladders rather than chairs or stools to reach high-up cabinets. When you're off balance, gravity generally wins," he says.

Make it stick, Slick. Give traction to high-traffic areas like hardwood floor walkways and especially hardwood stairs, suggests Taylor.

Also, if you haven't already, shell out the $1.99 and stick down some of those decorative, and potentially lifesaving, bathtub treads. The bathtub is a dangerous place to fall because you risk falling on something hard that provides no cushioning, warns Taylor.

Learn from Jackie. Try though you may, sometimes you just can't avoid life's little trip wires. By learning how to fall, you may be able to avoid the consequences of the tumble. Quintessential fall guy and martial arts mega star Jackie Chan has three key rules for hitting the ground safely.

1. Protect your head and back. When you feel yourself going down, try to land on your shoulders, thighs, and feet. Wrap your arms around your body to cushion the blow.
2. Don't fall on your head. A no-brainer!
3. Roll with it. If you use the momentum of the fall to keep rolling, instead of just hitting the ground with a thud, you'll lessen your chances of really hurting yourself.

Fire!

Despite all the warnings and public service announcements, fires and burns continue to be a leading cause of unintentional-injury deaths in U.S. homes. According to the National Fire Prevention Association (NFPA), fires currently cause about 4,700 deaths a year—nearly 4,000 (80 percent) of which are in the home. "Too often people mistakenly think that home fires are something that happen to someone else," says Susan McKelvey of the NFPA.

Maybe it's all those years spent playing fireman, but men in particular have a tendency to overestimate their fire safety knowledge, says McKelvey.

"Our most recent survey shows that though 63 percent of men said they felt confident about fire safety, twice as many men as women die in fires," McKelvey says. "The first and foremost rule when it comes to fire is, don't be a hero. Get out of the house and stay out." Even better, prevent fires in the first place. Here is what the NFPA recommends.

Carry a spoon. The largest cause of home fires in the United States is cooking, says McKelvey. "You're cooking. The phone rings. You leave the kitchen and forget all about your cooking. Next thing you know you smell smoke and return to find a fire. This type of scenario happens quite frequently," she says. Never leave cooking unattended, but if you need to leave the kitchen, carry a kitchen spoon or spatula with you to remind you that something's on the stove or in the oven, McKelvey suggests.

Keep a mitt on hand. Here's a simple but highly effective fire-prevention tactic. Keep an oven mitt that covers your arm by the stove along with a pot lid that fits the pan you are cooking with. That way, if those sweet potato fries go up in flames, you can quickly slide a mitt on your hand and a lid over that fire, says McKelvey. Then turn off the stove and let the pan cool completely. Don't lift the lid or you might re-ignite the flame, she says.

Flush that cigar. The kitchen may be the biggest hot spot in the house, but according to the NFPA, fires caused by careless smoking kill more than 800 people a year. The classic no-no, of course, is smoking in bed. You know not to do that. What you need to watch is how you dispose of cigarettes and cigars. "Too often, people think that their smoking materials are extinguished, they throw them out, and the hot

butts smolder for hours, eventually causing a fire in the middle of the night," McKelvey says. "The best practice is dousing cigarette butts thoroughly before discarding them by flushing ashtray contents down the toilet. Be especially aware of how your guests dispose of cigar and cigarette butts, particularly at parties where people are often drinking and not paying close attention."

Separate flammables. A simple reminder: Keep all combustible materials such as paint thinners and oils in sealed metal containers away from heat sources, says McKelvey. "Garages and basements are potential fire hazards."

Hang those detectors. Finally, install at least one smoke detector on every level of your home and in or near every sleeping area, McKelvey says. "Test them once a month and replace the battery annually. Having smoke detectors in your home cuts your chance of dying in a fire nearly in half," she says. And to make sure that you remember to change the batteries in those babies every year, tie the battery-changing to an annual event, such as your birthday, or when you set the clocks forward or back in the spring or fall.

A Shock to the System

Electrical shocks aren't the most common form of home accident, says Taylor. But they can be among the most harmful. "Even mild electrical shocks can result in serious internal injuries," adds Dr. Alton Thygerson of Brigham Young University and the National Safety Council's First-Aid Institute. "Even standard household current of 110 volts can be deadly."

The most basic way to avoid getting an unwanted shock to your system is to make it a cardinal rule not to mess with the wiring in your house unless you're a trained professional, Taylor says. "Be especially careful when you're drilling," he adds. "You don't want to be drilling around places where there could be electrical wires present, like outlets. When in doubt, always call an electrician. Your life is more important than the ego boost of doing it yourself."

If you do receive a shock, seek medical attention immediately, Dr. Thygerson says. "The burns on the skin that result from an electrical shock often are small and don't look like much, but electricity travels along your nerves and blood vessels before exiting your body. And even relatively minor shocks can cause internal damage."

Yardwork Woes

Your home doesn't end when you walk out the door. If you're like most homeowners, you likely have a patch of green—or more often stubbornly brown—that you call home for cookouts and lazy Sunday lounges. If you thought the inside of your house was an accident zone, check out what awaits in the backyard. The following are common yard-improvement tools, along with the number of handymen they send to the emergency room each year.

Nails, screws, and tacks or bolts:	191,037
Ladders:	151,327
Fences and fence posts:	114,055
Pruners, trimmers, and edgers:	36,204
Chain saws:	35,132
Gasoline and other fuels:	18,924
Pliers, wire cutters, and wrenches:	14,543

"Just like accidents that happen inside the house, accidents that happen in the yard are often the result of cutting corners or being overly confident," Taylor says. The following tips can help.

Cover up. "We tell people that if they're

Check, Please

Think your home is a safe haven? Go through this quick checklist compiled by Lowe's Home Safety Council and the National Safety Council to find out.

Does your home have:

Smoke detectors? Install them on every level, including the basement and outside all sleeping areas. Test the batteries once a month.

A carbon monoxide (CO) detector? Any fuel-burning appliance is a potential source of this deadly gas. Be sure to have at least one CO detector near your sleeping areas.

Ground-fault circuit interrupters (GFCIs)? GFCIs monitor the electricity flowing to a circuit, shutting it off if an imbalance occurs. They should be placed on circuits to the bathrooms, laundry rooms, kitchens, swimming pools, and outdoor receptacles. Test them monthly.

Fire extinguishers? Mount a multipurpose dry chemical class 2A:10B:C fire extinguisher near the main exits of each level of your home so that, in case of fire, a person using the extinguisher can easily escape the house if the fire spreads. Teach yourself and your family when and how to use it properly.

An emergency evacuation plan? You should have at least two exits from every room in the house and practice each escape route from the house with everyone in your home.

Flashlights? Keep 'em stocked with fresh batteries at all bedsides and in the basement.

A first-aid kit? Make sure that everyone knows where it is, what's in it, and how and when to use it.

Emergency phone numbers? Include police, fire, doctors, and poison-control centers. Post them at every telephone in the house.

Tagged shutoffs? Place tags on your home shutoff valves for gas, oil, water, and the main electrical supply when you turn them off to work on them so that no one accidentally turns them back on.

going to be working around the old house, take their cue from Bob Vila or Norm Abram," says Taylor. "They always wear gloves and safety goggles and take the little precautions that can

Grab bars? **Install grab bars in all bathtubs and shower stalls.**

Slip-resistant finishes? **Use a nonskid mat, or install strips or decals in bathtubs or showers.**

Safety glazing? **Any glass paneling in your home, including shower doors, patio doors, or window walls, should be made with safety glass.**

Handrails? **Every set of stairs should have handrails securely mounted to both sides of the stairs.**

A stepstool/utility ladder? **Keep one handy to prevent you from climbing up on a chair when you need to get to hard-to-reach places.**

Sufficient lighting? **Use night-lights near bathrooms, bedrooms, and stairwells. Keep stairs and hallways well-lit. Provide adequate lighting to all walkways and entrances to your home.**

Tested appliances? **All electric and gas appliances should carry an Underwriters Laboratories (UL), Canadian Standards Association (CSA), or American Gas Association (AGA) label on them.**

Safety goggles? **Safety goggles or safety glasses are essential for home improvement work.**

A survival kit? **In case of natural disasters, have a kit that includes tools, a battery-operated radio, flashlight, clothing and bedding, water, nonperishable food, and a first-aid kit.**

Childproofing? **Include cabinet locks for poisons and medicines, outlet covers, safety gates for stairs, fireplace screens, spout guards and a bathtub mixer faucet for hot and cold water, edge guards for sharp edges on furniture and fireplace hearths, and protective surfacing in play areas.**

Swimming pool safety? **Pools should have a four-foot fence with a self-closing, self-latching gate, life preservers, rescue equipment, a lockable storage space for chemicals, and a poolside telephone.**

Take your time. Whatever you do, don't rush yourself on a domestic-repair or improvement job. Haste can waste you. "The worst thing you can do," Taylor says, "is not allow yourself enough time to do the job properly. Many accidents occur when you try to do too much in too little time." If you really don't have time to do the job right, get somebody else to do it—like a professional—or don't do it at all.

Building a Safe House

Though the vast majority of accidents are preventable, sometimes bad things happen in good homes. A generally reliable coal burner starts leaking carbon monoxide. Electrical appliances short circuit. Bad moons rise and disasters strike. Though you can't always foresee or prevent an incident from occurring, you can set up your home to launch counterstrikes should one start, says Taylor. "The key is arming your home with all the proper safety devices like carbon monoxide detectors, fire extinguishers, first-aid kits, and the like."

Finally, aside from prevention, the very best thing you can do for yourself and your family is learn how to treat accidents when they happen, says Heather McMurtrie, senior associate of health and safety services at the American Red Cross national headquarters in Washington, D.C. "We recommend that everybody get trained in basic first-aid and CPR (cardiopulmonary resuscitation). You can enroll in a class by calling your local Red Cross chapter," she says. Just look for the number in the white pages of your phone book. Or write to the National Safety Council First-Aid Institute, 1121 Spring Lake Drive, Itasca, IL 60143-3201, for classes in your area.

keep you out of big trouble." It's especially important to take these safety precautions when handling power equipment, like mowers and pruners.

Accidents at Work

Falling Down on the Job

Every day, 17 people go to their death after going to work. Each year, more than 6,000 people are killed on the job—92 percent of whom are men. And you thought your *home* life was stressful?

As you might expect, those at greatest risk for dying on the job are men who work in the great outdoors, where the whims of Mother Nature often become a factor, says Guy A. Toscano, economist in the Office of Safety, Health, and Working Conditions at the Bureau of Labor Statistics in Washington, D.C. Fishermen and loggers have it the worst by far. While the national average for deaths on the job is 5 out of every 100,000 workers, these outdoorsmen die at rates 20 to 30 times higher—losing more than 100 workers and, in some years, even rates as high as 150, out of every 100,000 on the job. "Truck drivers, farmers, and construction laborers have occupations that have high fatality rates as well as high numbers of job-related fatal injuries as well," says Toscano.

But as bad as those figures sound, things are actually better than they used to be. Back in 1912, when we knew (and some would say cared) less about job safety, between 18,000 and 21,000 workers a year lost their lives while earning their daily bread. By 1995, with a work force more than triple in size producing 13 times as many goods and services, occupational deaths had decreased by more than two-thirds. "We have be-

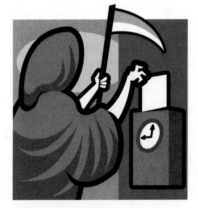

come more aware of safety issues in society at large," explains Michael Buchet, manager of the construction division and the labor division at the National Safety Council in Itasca, Illinois. "In industry, we've been encouraging safer workplace practices and are pushing for training, training, and more training."

That said, after decades of progress, it seems harder to make gains in workplace safety these days, Toscano says. "We've clearly hit a plateau in that the number of fatal occupational injuries has held steady at the 6,000 to 6,500 mark for the past five years," he says. "That doesn't mean that we can't make any more progress. But it does mean that safety professionals have to be willing to work harder to recognize risk and promote safety measures."

Risky Business

The first thing to understand is that some occupations are hazardous by virtue of the type of work. And you'd better know an occupation's risks when you get into it so that you can either take extra precautions or choose a safer line of work, says Toscano. Take elephant training, for example. Some years, the elephants get testy or trainers are careless or lack training, and one or two trainers are killed. Because there are only about 600 elephant trainers in the United States to begin with, having one or two killed during a single year can make it one of the riskiest occupations—with a fatal injury rate 68 times higher than that of the average American worker.

Sure, elephant training is an extreme example. But consider that every day, thousands of men face jobs almost as dangerous as teaching Jumbo to sit.

Chances are that if you've ever thought about giving it all up to live off the land (or the sea, for those who fancy the water), you've never actually tried it. Farms look bucolic.

Forests seem peaceful. Seas appear serene. But making a living as a farmer, woodsman, or fisherman is not only hard work; it can be downright deadly.

In 1995, the most recent year for which data have been analyzed, farm occupations were the 10th most fatal in the nation, with a rate of 25.3 deaths a year for every 100,000 workers; 579 were killed that year. Tractor-related incidents—including rollovers, falls, and highway collisions—are responsible for about one out of every three farm-related deaths. Twelve farmers a year on average are killed by angry farm animals. Plus, farmers face lightning strikes, heatstroke, bee stings, razor-sharp farm equipment, and often severe weather conditions.

Folks in the timber and logging industry don't have it any better. At a rate of 101 out of every 100,000 timber cutters dying on the job, timber and logging is the second most deadly occupation in the nation. Of the 98 timber cutters who were killed in 1995, 82 percent were struck by falling trees.

Finally, taking your livelihood to the seas is literally taking your life into your hands. With a rate of 104.4 docksiders dying for every 100,000 folks who hoist nets and poles for a living, fishing is the most dangerous occupation in the country today. Not surprising, the leading cause of fishing fatalities is drowning.

If you're seeking safer employment, try a job in an industry like service and finance, insurance or real estate, where only about 2 out of every 100,000 people are killed at work each year. Otherwise, if you're one of the legion of laborers who risk life and limb every day to get the job done, experts recommend taking a long, hard look at what kills people in your field and

Cops and Jobbers

If you were to judge by the TV show, nobody has it worse than cops when it comes to fatal occupations. In reality, though, being a cab driver carries almost three times the risk of walking the beat. Both occupations have the highest risk of becoming a homicide victim while working. Here are the 10 deadliest jobs in the United States today, according to Bureau of Labor Statistics. The risk index compares fatality for a given group of workers to the overall rate for all workers. In plain English: The higher the index, the deadlier the job.

Occupation	1995 Fatalities	Total Number of Employees	Risk Index	Leading Fatal Event
All workers	6,210	126,246,000	1.0	Highway crashes
1. Fishermen	48	45,000	21.3	Drowning
2. Timber cutters	98	97,000	20.6	Struck by object (example: falling trees)
3. Aircraft pilots	111	114,000	19.9	Aircraft crashes
4. Structural metal workers	38	59,000	13.1	Falling
5. Taxicab drivers	99	213,000	9.5	Homicide
6. Construction laborers	309	780,000	8.1	Vehicular accidents and falling
7. Roofers	60	205,000	5.9	Falling
8. Electrical installation/repair	35	126,000	5.7	Electrocution
9. Truck drivers	749	2.9 million	5.3	Highway crashes
10. Farm occupations	579	2.3 million	5.1	Vehicular accidents

SOURCE: U.S. Department of Labor, Bureau of Labor Statistics, Census of Fatal Occupational Injuries, 1995; published in "Dangerous Jobs," *Compensation and Working Conditions*, 1997.

taking precautions to make sure that you live to work another day. Here's what labor experts have to say about some the nation's deadliest occupations.

Truckin'

Truck driving ranks ninth on the list of lethal jobs and accounts for more job-related deaths than any other occupation—killing 749 drivers in 1995, or 13 percent of all job-related deaths. Of those fatalities, 68 percent are a direct result of highway crashes. That means that every day, at least one truck driver is killed in a highway vehicle crash. But there's a lot that drivers and their employers can do to make things safer for themselves, their employees, and the rest of us on the road.

Maintain a safe limit. One of the most likely culprits behind the increased incidence of fatalities in the transportation industry is the increased speed limits in many states. According to Department of Transportation statistics, when speed limits increase, so do highway fatalities.

Embrace new technology. Truck drivers are supposed to keep logs to ensure that they aren't pushing themselves too hard and driving with too little sleep. But logs mean very little, and some safety professionals instead recommend using smart technology for trucks. For example, devices are available that monitor the number of hours a truck is running.

Train and maintain. One of the simplest ways to reduce trucker highway fatalities is to promote driver training programs and proper vehicle maintenance. Both of these are too essential to be skimped on in the name of cost savings.

The Hard-Hat Zone

When Joseph B. Strauss designed and engineered America's second-largest bridge

across the Golden Gate Strait, he was determined that this San Francisco project would be the safest in bridge-construction history. Local safety equipment manufacturer Edward W. Bullard developed the first "hard hat," workers were fed a special diet to prevent dizziness, and a safety net was suspended below the floor of the bridge from end to end. That net saved a total of 19 men, proving that safety measures worked. Then in 1937, a few months before the bridge was to open, a section of scaffold carrying 12 men fell and ripped through the safety net, killing 10 of them—proving also that construction was, is, and likely always will be inherently dangerous.

Today, falls remain a leading cause of death and disability at construction sites. In one year alone, it's common to have more than 40,000 disabling falls. When those falls happen from roofs, scaffolding, or other temporary platforms, workers often don't get back up. Making matters on the construction site even worse are vehicular accidents and electrocutions, which account for almost as many fatalities as falls.

With more than 309 deaths in 1995—or a rate of 39.5 for every 100,000 workers—being a construction laborer ranks as the sixth deadliest occupation in the United States. No doubt, we're always going to need bridges and buildings, but we need to keep our construction workers safe, says Toscano. Here's what experts recommend.

Strap on protection. There is no shortage of products on the market to help prevent a construction worker's fall, Toscano says. "Some fasten the workers to a stable part of the construction site. Some work like a seat belt and 'catch' the worker should he suddenly slip." But according to some safety professionals, many of the daredevils in these fields don't want to wear them. For example, roofers have actually fought to be exempt from fall-protection regulations because they maintain that the equipment contributes to falls rather than preventing them.

Work along the curve.

"Being new on a job increases your chances for getting hurt," Buchet says. "The newness of the work, the lighting, and the conditions all put you at risk when you start a job, no matter what your age. It's best to be aware of that and respect your learning curve."

White-Collar Woes

If you're among the legion of button-down desk jockeys or other nonlaborers in the workforce, you don't have to worry much about death by toppling trees or by falling hundreds of feet from scaffolding. Your co-workers are another story. One in three workplaces has been the site of a violent episode. Every day two or three workers are fatally shot at work.

Assaults and violent acts comprise 20 percent of fatal occupational injuries. When they happen at work, your employer takes a certain amount of responsibility for them and they are logged as occupational "intentional deaths"—the safety industry's word for not being an accident. Right now, getting shot is the biggest risk for some white-collar workers, Toscano says.

"Though this occupational risk seems more out of the victim's control than, say, strapping on a safety belt, that doesn't mean that you're helpless from preventing these events from occurring," adds Toscano. "For example, I can remember back in the 1970s, anybody could just walk into the federal building where I worked. But circumstances have changed. Now we have employee identification and access cards to restrict entrance of potential perpetrators of violent acts in the workplace.

"If your workplace seems vulnerable to

Working Yourself to Death

Since the time of ancient Egypt, when men routinely lost their lives hauling millions of two-ton stone blocks to erect the Great Egyptian Pyramids, men have been literally working themselves to death. The following are how some of today's industries stack up in the fatality department.

Industry	Number (Occupational Fatalities)	Percent (of Total Occupational Fatalities)	Rate per 100,000 Workers
Total (1995)	6,210	100	5
Agriculture, forestry, and fishing	793	13	22
Mining and quarrying	156	3	25
Construction	1,048	17	15
Manufacturing	702	11	3
Transportation and public utilities	880	14	12
Wholesale trade	254	4	5
Retail trade	675	11	3
Finance, insurance, and real estate	124	2	2
Services	737	12	2
Government*	772	12	4

*Includes fatalities to workers employed by government organizations regardless of industry.
SOURCE: U.S. Department of Labor, Bureau of Labor Statistics, Census of Fatal Occupational Injuries.
NOTE: Percentages may not add to totals because of rounding. There were 69 fatalities for which there was insufficient information to determine specific industry classification.

outside invasion, safety experts suggest that your employer install a security system, especially if your job involves handling money. Employers often take these suggestions seriously," says Toscano.

Accidents at Play

Out for the Count

It seems like we'll do anything for kicks. Careen down rocky mountain trails on a bicycle? You bet. Strap skis to our feet and get dragged behind a boat? Sounds like a blast. Surprisingly (and fortunately), as reckless and dangerous as the activities we call sport may sound, they don't often kill us. More often, they just beat the crap out of us.

Plenty of weekend warriors are injured in sports like basketball, bicycling, football, and softball. They're rarely deadly, but collectively, they report astronomical injury rates, which is where the trouble really lies. We hardly have to tell you that, even if injuries don't kill you, they can sure take their toll on your body over time. And serious injuries, such as those to the head, neck, or back, can cause permanent debilitating problems like brain damage and paralysis.

"That's why we encourage people to take just a few minor precautions during their recreational activities," says Dr. Jeffrey Sacks of the National Center for Injury Prevention and Control.

By following a few basic rules, you can put your safest foot forward next time you step out to play.

Put the beer on ice. Alcohol is an enormous factor in recreational injuries, Dr. Sacks says. So don't be stupid. "When you're drowning from a waterskiing incident because you're drunk, that's no accident. That's preventable. Save the beer for afterward," says Dr. Sacks.

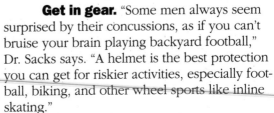

Get in gear. "Some men always seem surprised by their concussions, as if you can't bruise your brain playing backyard football," Dr. Sacks says. "A helmet is the best protection you can get for riskier activities, especially football, biking, and other wheel sports like inline skating."

Take charge. We have a whole industry devoted to "adventure travel" where people do relatively risky activities rather safely, says Dr. Alton Thygerson of Brigham Young University and the National Safety Council's First-Aid Institute. "That's because the folks in charge know what they're doing. You can help prevent being another accident statistic by learning the fundamentals of an activity before you start, especially ones that involve some risk like water sports or mountain biking."

Spinning Safely

In 1992, men made up the overwhelming majority of bike fatalities—almost 90 percent, with the death rate for men on bikes being nearly seven times that of female spinners. Why? "Why else?" says Dr. Sacks. "Men push the envelope more, sometimes when they shouldn't." To stay safer in the saddle, especially on the road where traffic is an issue, the National Highway Traffic Safety Administration recommends heeding these fundamental cycling rules.

Put a lid on it. Buy a helmet that complies with standards of the American National Standards Institute (ANSI) or Snell Memorial Foundation (SNELL)—it should say so on the label—and, more important, wear the darn thing. Bike helmets reduce head injuries by 85 percent. Your helmet's side straps should meet in a "V" just below your ears. It shouldn't shift when you shake your head.

Stay bright. Bike clothes come in wild colors for a reason: so that you can be seen. Always wear neon or fluorescent colors when cycling.

Be a day-tripper. Well over a third of fatal bike accidents occur during the hard-to-see dusk hours of 4:00 P.M. to 8:00 P.M. Riding after dark is even more dangerous. If you must ride after the sun sets, get a bicycle light and wear reflective cycling clothing.

Ride right. Ride on the right side with the flow of traffic, single file, and signal when you're going to turn.

Check traffic. More than 70 percent of car-bicycle accidents happen at intersections and driveways. Obey traffic laws such as stop signs and traffic lights, and always be alert for traffic.

Smooth Sailing

As the number of personal watercrafts (PWCs), especially Jet Skis and Waverunners, increases on our nation's waterways, so does the number of men who are injuring or killing themselves in accidents. In just five years, the annual injury rate from PWCs skyrocketed from 532 per year to 1,338. To keep yourself sailing more smoothly and safely, the National Association of State Boating Law Administrators suggests the following steps.

Keep afloat. Always wear a life jacket. "That way, even if you hurt yourself in a crash, you can stay afloat," says Dr. Thygerson.

Take a course. Boating associations recommend that everyone, even Jet Ski operators, take a safe-boating course to learn safety regulations, the traffic laws of the water, and proper PWC operation.

Play Hard

When it comes to sports, it seems like nothing's safe. Check out the following list of popular recreational activities and their annual injury totals.

Sport	Participants	Injuries
Baseball, softball	33,300,000	366,064
Basketball	30,100,000	692,396
Bicycle riding (mountain and road)	72,500,000	586,808
Billiards, pool	31,100,000	4,484
Bowling	41,900,000	22,224
Exercising with equipment (including weight lifting)	44,300,000	86,157
Fishing	44,200,000	80,515
Football	20,400,000	389,463
Golf (excluding golf cart injuries)	24,000,000	39,247
Roller skating (inline and side-by-side)	37,500,000	175,295
Soccer	12,000,000	156,960
Swimming	61,500,000	134,022
Tennis	12,600,000	25,934
Volleyball	18,000,000	86,551

SOURCES: Participants—National Sporting Goods Association (1995); figures include those who participate more than one time per year except for bicycle riding and swimming, which include those who participate more than six times per year. Injuries—Consumer Product Safety Commission (1995); figures include only injuries treated in hospital emergency rooms.

Ski Smart

You don't have to crash head over heels like the guy in the "agony of defeat" sequence from the opening of *ABC's Wide World of Sports* to do some permanent damage on the slopes. "You just have to have a poorly executed fall. Or hit something, like a tree," Dr. Sacks says. Proper precautions can avoid many of these injuries, says Dr. Thygerson. If you're considering trying a new snow sport like snowboarding or would like to be more daring on your skis, take an advanced lesson.

Suicide

The Real Silent Killer

For the past 50 years or so, we've been killing ourselves with a silent bang. It's a little-known fact that suicide is the ninth leading cause of death in this country and the fifth leading cause among men ages 25 to 44.

There is no simple answer for why men commit suicide, says John L. McIntosh, Ph.D., professor of psychology at Indiana University in South Bend, who works with the American Association of Suicidology in Washington, D.C.

The Depression Connection

Nearly 95 percent of people who kill themselves are suffering from a psychiatric illness—most often depression—in the months before they commit suicide. Yet, it often goes undiagnosed, says Matthew Nock, research coordinator for the American Foundation for Suicide Prevention (AFSP) in New York City.

To be fair, detection is difficult because men often don't let on that they're in trouble, at least not in obvious ways, Dr. McIntosh says. Men also may have underlying biological tendencies for self-destruction that we just don't understand yet, say suicide researchers. For one, men have lower levels of the brain neurotransmitter serotonin than women. And not only are people with low levels of this mood-governing chemical prone to depression but also research suggests that their suicide risk is 10 times that of people with higher levels.

And that's not the only chemical connection. Very low cholesterol levels—less than 160

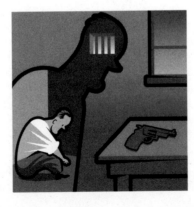

milligrams per deciliter—have also been linked to elevated suicide risk in men. Researchers in Paris found that of more than 6,000 men they studied, those with low cholesterol levels were more than three times more likely to commit suicide during the four-year study than those with normal cholesterol levels.

Drinking and drug use seem to add mental anguish all their own, says Dr. McIntosh. Alcoholism is a factor in 30 percent of all completed suicides. And cocaine ranks right up there with depression and alcohol abuse as a primary risk factor.

Personal loss, particularly of a wife or a job, is another leading factor. For every rise in the divorce rate (measured as one extra divorce per 1,000 couples), there is a 35 percent increase in male suicide rates. And men without jobs commit suicide twice as often as men who have them.

Illness, Aging, and Genes

Two other suicide hot spots include sickness and old age, which are often, but certainly not always, synonymous. And there also may be a genetic link, experts say.

Men ages 20 to 59 who have been diagnosed with AIDS, for instance, are about 36 times more likely to commit suicide than men of the same age who do not have the disease. Barring diseases such as AIDS, however, the older you get, the greater your chances for getting seriously ill, and the greater your risk for suicide.

Medical illness is a direct contributor to suicide in up to 70 percent of all suicide victims older than 60. White men over 50 are especially vulnerable. Though they make up only 10 percent of the population, this volatile group is responsible for a third of all suicides.

Yet doctors have found that, like other suicidal people, those who wish to die while they are ill most often are suffering not from a pain-induced, well-pondered death wish but from clinical depression or alcoholism. When their depression is treated, they usually don't want to die any longer, according to the AFSP.

Like your height and eye color, suicidal tendencies are unfortunately passed on along family lines. If someone in your family has killed himself, your risk of doing the same increases fourfold.

There are a couple of reasons for this, say AFSP researchers. First, there may be an actual biological-suicidal characteristic that is inherited, such as the inability to process serotonin correctly. Second, families don't just share genes; they share environments, says Dr. McIntosh. "We live with the same stressful situations. And if you see your parents acting out in a certain way, you're likely to pick up that behavior, no matter how destructive."

Following the Signs

Though a few suicides occur out of the blue, 75 percent of people who attempt suicide give some warning to their friends and family, Nock says. You should become familiar with the primary danger signs that signal someone is contemplating suicide, says Nock. They are:

- Previous suicide attempts. Trying to kill yourself once is one of the best predictors of whether you'll actually take your life one day. Between 20 percent and 50 percent of people who kill themselves have tried before.
- Talking about death. People who commit suicide often talk about death. Sometimes they say goodbye or act as though they're going away.
- Making final arrangements. Suicidal people often go about putting their af-

---

Suicide States

According to statistics from the American Association of Suicidology, maybe the traffic-ridden, congested northeastern states aren't so bad after all. Check out the states with the highest and lowest suicide rates and judge for yourself.

State	Rate per 100,000 People	Number
High-Risk		
1. Nevada	25.8	395
2. Montana	23.1	201
3. Arizona	19.1	805
4. New Mexico	17.6	297
5. Colorado	17.5	654
Low-Risk		
1. Washington, D.C.	7	39
2. New Jersey	7.3	578
3. New York	7.6	1,370
4. Massachusetts	8.1	489
5. Rhode Island	9	89

NOTE: Suicide rates are calculated by dividing the number of suicides among a group by the number of people in the group and multiplying that by 100,000. This allows researchers to compare suicide rates among groups of differing populations. The number of suicides given is simply the number of "successful" suicides in one year.

---

fairs in order as though they have a terminal illness. They may give away possessions or pay off large debts or mortgages.

- Showing signs of depression. Be especially concerned if people withdraw from activities they used to enjoy or have changes in sleeping patterns, appetite, weight, energy, or sex drive. These, along with feelings of worthlessness and thoughts of death, are signs of depression.

If you recognize these in yourself or another, check your local listings for a suicide prevention hotline.

Homicide

Staying Safe on the Mean Streets

In 1995, more than 21,500 people were murdered in America. That's about 8 out of every 100,000 people. Homicide is the second leading cause of death among all young people ages 15 to 24. What's more, 77 percent of the people killed in 1995 were men.

Yet the reality is that violent crime is on the decline. During the past five years or so, violent crimes such as assault and battery have dropped about 12.4 percent. The murder rate itself has dropped 13 percent. So why do we still feel so unsafe?

The Smoking Gun

Ask most cops how to cut down on homicide and they'll give you two words: "gun control." Eight out of every 10 murders are committed with a gun, most often a handgun.

Contrary to the message sent by the John Waynes and Dirty Harrys out there, packing your own heat is not the solution to gun violence, says Hubert Williams, president of the Police Foundation in Washington, D.C. "The great majority of people who get guns are not trained to use them, and that doesn't just mean how to fire them," says Williams, who was a police director in Newark, New Jersey, for 11 years. "Your chances of getting shot by someone who has a gun on you is much higher if you have a gun, too. Plus, too often the perpetrator doesn't have a weapon until he gets his hands on yours."

And that's not even considering how risky it is just to have a gun in your house. A firearm in your home is 40 times more likely to hurt or kill you or a family member than it is to stop a crime, says the National Crime Prevention Council (NCPC), in Washington, D.C.

There are better ways to protect yourself against gun violence, says Williams. Here's what he recommends.

Take up the arts. "If I had to name one effective form of self-defense for almost everybody, it would be the martial arts," Williams says. Not just because they teach you how to throw a kick or a punch, but because you learn a mental discipline that teaches you how to handle potentially violent conflicts without getting hurt. You also learn to develop the presence of mind to sense dangerous situations before you get into them, he says.

Take a stand. To keep guns from the hands of folks who shouldn't have them, continue to support laws like the Brady Bill that require background checks for purchasing a firearm. The Bureau of Justice Statistics reported that since the Brady Bill took effect in 1994, 173,000 illegal handgun sales—meaning sales to someone with a criminal record—have been blocked.

It's Who You Know

You've likely heard it before, but we'll tell you again. If you gather all the homicide statistics and extract drug-related homicides, the vast majority of murders are between people who know each other. Forty-four percent of people who are murdered are killed by someone they know.

Obviously, that doesn't mean that you should start looking at your golf buddies askance, but do be careful whom you make serious acquaintance with, says Jean O'Neil, director of research and policy at the NCPC. "And certainly use some discretion when it comes to whom you hang out with, even casually," she says.

The following can help you check for potentially dangerous liaisons.

Inspect the fuse. "Not to liken people to canines, but you know which dogs are likely to bite and which are not by their mannerisms," Williams says. "People are the same way. If someone is hostile and aggressive or, worse, has acted violently in the past, even if it wasn't toward you, don't get involved with them. These are folks with short fuses who are capable of hurting you, too, if you upset them." If you doubt the seriousness of this situation, consider that 28 percent of murders occur as the result of an argument, according to the FBI.

Just say no. "People who are serious drug users are another group to avoid," says Williams, "especially if they seem pretty solid until they're high or drunk and then get mean. That can indicate a dangerous person." Statistics show that he's right. Almost half of all violent offenders serving time in state prisons have admitted to being under the influence of drugs or alcohol when they committed their crimes.

Home, Sweet Home

"Homicide is a public health risk like any other," says Williams. "Just like you can lower your cancer risk by not smoking, you can lower your risk of homicide by living and hanging out in safer places." Here's how to check out your own locale.

Call the police. The simplest way to tell whether a neighborhood you want to move into is safe is by calling the local police and asking for someone in the crime prevention or

States of Violence	
Looking for that safe haven? Here are some states that may qualify and a few that, well, may not, based on the FBI Uniform Crime Reports for 1995.	
State	Number of Murders per 100,000
The Best	
North Dakota	0.9
Iowa	1.8
New Hampshire	1.8
South Dakota	1.8
Wyoming	2.1
The Worst	
Washington, D.C.	65
Louisiana	17
Mississippi	12.9
Oklahoma	12.2
California	11.2

community affairs office. Also, talk to neighbors and local business owners, says O'Neil. You'll be able to find out about crime in the town or even on your particular street.

Sign up. Your current or potential neighborhood probably also has a local crime watch group, says O'Neil. These can be useful not just for finding out crime statistics but in curtailing crime as well. Getting involved also introduces you to people in the neighborhood who can keep an eye out for you and your home.

Use your head. Finally, the best way to prevent becoming a victim of homicide is to use your head, says the NCPC. Whether you're on the street or in your car, you should always be alert to your surroundings. Project a calm, confident attitude. Trust your instincts; if something or someone doesn't feel right, they probably aren't. Know the neighborhoods surrounding where you live and work. And by all means, if someone tries to rob you, give up the material stuff, says the NCPC. It's not worth your life.

Acts of God

Expecting the Unexpected

Drive your car into a tree and it's an act of stupidity. Put a patch of ice under your tires and suddenly it's God's fault. Though scientists hate the phrase "act of God," everyday folks have been blaming not-so-everyday disasters like twisters, blizzards, and floods on random acts of the divine since Noah picked up his first two-by-four. The government has officially recognized acts of God as a public health concern since the 1600s. Insurance companies use the phrase to describe just about any major disaster. But the fact is that most of us are still as unprepared for sudden disaster as the folks who didn't make it onto the ark.

"A lot of people have some of the things they need for a crisis, but since they never really think it'll happen to them, they aren't prepared to the extent they should be," explains Nina Johnson, disaster manager at the American Red Cross, Lehigh Valley Chapter, in Bethlehem, Pennsylvania. "And that can cause big problems when disasters strike."

Hurricanes, tornadoes, snowstorms, and the like kill about 245 people each year, according to National Safety Council statistics. "And though these events are often unexpected, that doesn't mean that they have to be unanticipated," says Mary Hudak, public information officer for the Federal Emergency Management Agency in Atlanta. The state and federal governments have great systems in place to help you out in times of crisis, but to survive, you need to educate yourself about your risk and be well-prepared. That means being able to survive 72 hours without assistance, and often electricity. Here's what you need to know.

Winter Storm Warnings

Just two blizzards—the first in March 1993, the second in January 1996—combined to claim the lives of 300 people in the eastern United States. And the majority of those who die in winter storms are men over 40. With the National Weather Service's ability to predict storms well in advance, there's really little excuse for letting Old Man Winter knock you out for the count. Next time, take these steps.

Take warning. "The most important thing is to listen to the watches and warnings," Johnson says. "Watches mean that a storm *could* happen. A warning means that it will. A blizzard warning means that it's going to be big. Watches change to warnings very quickly, so when you hear a watch, make sure that you stock up on the essentials like food, diapers, bottled water, and anything else you need."

Get off the road. Seventy percent of ice- and snow-related winter deaths happen in cars, according to the American Red Cross. If you must go out, the organization recommends carrying a disaster supply kit in your car and filling your gas tank frequently to keep the fuel lines from freezing. If you get stuck, stay with your car. Just run the engine for 10 minutes every hour with the dome light on for visibility; crack a window to let some air in, and tie a bright cloth to your antenna.

Take shelter. Seventy-five percent of people who die from cold exposure are men. Stay inside, if possible. If you must go out, wear many loose-fitting layers of clothes, covered by a tightly woven, water-repellent coat. Cover your mouth with scarves to protect your lungs from the cold air, says Johnson.

Work lightly. "All the snow does not have to be cleared from your sidewalks within one hour after a snowfall," Johnson says. Cold weather puts a strain on your heart, so regardless of your age or physical condition, you can have a heart attack while shoveling snow. Take frequent breaks.

When the Earth Moves

Over the past decade, two powerful earthquakes have rocked California, collectively killing 119 people, injuring more than 12,500, and costing more than $19 billion in damages. Geographers say that the odds are 67 percent that another large earthquake will shake the San Francisco Bay area within the next 30 years. Though California is at greatest risk, no state is immune. You can't buy a crystal ball to tell you when or where the next earthquake will hit, but you can take action to protect yourself, should one hit close to home.

Duck, cover, and hold. The old advice to stand in the doorway during an earthquake isn't particularly useful in modern houses since the doorways aren't very strong. Your best bet is to crawl under a sturdy piece of furniture and duck, cover, and hold on. Stay clear of windows, fireplaces, china cabinets, and heavy appliances, says Johnson.

Find a clearing. If you're outside, try to get as far away from buildings and power lines as possible. If you're in your car, stop driving, and park your car away from light posts, bridges, trees, and telephone poles, says Johnson.

Batten down the hatches. Fasten shelving to the walls, making sure that the fasteners go into wall studs. Fasten the TV and the stereo down. Strap large appliances such as stoves and refrigerators to a wall so that they don't fall over. Try to fix cabinets and cupboards so that they don't easily fly open and spill their contents, says Johnson.

Shut down. "If you're in a high-risk quake area, you need to know how to shut off

---

Do-It-Yourself Disaster Kit

It's much easier to gather everything you need for an emergency when nothing's wrong than when the flood waters are 10 feet high and rising, says Nina Johnson of the American Red Cross. Pack a disaster kit with the following basics. For a more detailed list, contact your local American Red Cross chapter.

- Three-day supply of water—each person gets one gallon per day
- Three-day supply of food, preferably canned meats, fruits, and vegetables (don't forget a manual can opener)
- First-aid supplies
- Warm clothing and bedding
- Tools and supplies, such as flashlights, maps, mess kits, battery-operated radio, matches, and a fire extinguisher
- Personal supplies, such as toilet paper and personal hygiene items

---

your gas," Hudak says. "You should also be prepared for a complete shutdown of your basic services like electricity and water. After an earthquake, fill your bathtub with the water remaining in the pipes so that you have water for sanitary uses if the main lines have broken."

Twister!

It's a myth that tornadoes "suck up" cows, small dogs, and houses into their funnel. So don't worry about becoming an accessory to the storm if a twister's heading your way. What you should worry about is getting struck by Bessie, Toto, or even a Toyota, because with winds in excess of 250 miles per hour, a tornado can lift and toss large objects hundreds of feet from its path. It can also leave a path of destruction 1 mile wide and 50 miles long, so it's best to take cover when a tornado blows into town. Here's how you can keep from twisting in the wind.

Stay tuned. "Doppler weather forecasters can locate a tornado before it touches down," says Johnson. Since tornadoes occur as the result of a nasty thunderstorm, you should check out the radio or television news if there's a bad boomer in your area. You also can buy a weather radio with a warning alarm that will turn on automatically and warn you when a tornado watch or warning has been issued. They are available at electronics stores.

Go when it's green. If you're out and about, be warned when the sky turns green, there's large hail, you see a wall of clouds, or you hear a loud roar like a freight train. These are signs that a tornado may be on the way—unless, of course, you live next to the railroad tracks.

Get down. "Get to the basement if you can," says Johnson. "If you can't, go to a center hallway, a bathroom, or a closet on the lowest floor. You want to find a strong, low location."

Get outta the car. If you're in your car or a mobile home during a tornado, get out and find shelter. If you can't get into the basement of a nearby building, lie flat in a ditch or low-lying area.

When the Levee Breaks

That mean old levee sure does make us weep and moan—especially when it breaks. Flash floods can happen anywhere there are streams and sewers. And in the time it takes to soft-boil an egg, rising flood waters can hit peaks of 30 feet or more. "Take flash flood warnings very seriously," warns

When Lightning Strikes

You're on the seventh hole, and you hear thunder in the distance. What do you do? None of the other players looks concerned, and this is your first day off in months. So you decide to play on. It's the smart thing to do, right?

Wrong. No one, not even a golfer, is immune to lightning. Lightning kills about 100 people a year, and injures hundreds more, says Michael Cherington, M.D., clinical professor of neurology at the University of Colorado School of Medicine and founder of the Lightning Data Center at Centura Health, both in Denver. Men are four times as likely to get jolted as women, perhaps, in part, because they don't come in out of the rain. He recommends several ways to lower your risk.

Pick up the signals. Darkening skies, sudden drops in temperature, and increasing wind are all pretty good signs that a storm is coming and you ought to head for cover.

Use your ears. If you can hear thunder, you're close enough to get zapped. You can measure how far away the storm is by counting seconds between the flash of lightning

Johnson. "You only have minutes or seconds to act."

Get high. A flood watch means that a flood is possible. A warning means that it's coming very soon. When you hear a watch, move your furniture and valuables to higher floors in your home and fill your gas tank. If you hear a warning, be ready to evacuate the area and find higher ground on a moment's notice, according to the American Red Cross.

Abandon ship. "If you're in your car, do not drive into the water. I don't care how shallow it looks," implores Johnson. Cars are easily swept away in just two feet of water. If the water's rising quickly around your car, get out and climb to higher ground.

and the thunder—every five seconds equals roughly one mile—but just seek safe shelter immediately.

Follow an 11:00 A.M. curfew. If you're hiking high altitudes like the Rocky Mountains, get down below timberline by 11:00 A.M., Dr. Cherington says. "Most strikes occur after this time during the day."

Seek safe shelter. The safest place during a storm is inside a safe shelter. When indoors, stay off the phone, out of the shower or bathtub, and away from appliances.

Stay away from single trees. If you're on a golf course or any other open area, do *not* seek refuge under an isolated tree. The inside of a closed car or van is a relatively safe place to be. If a vehicle or safe shelter is not nearby, run into a forest rather than under a single tree. If you're outside and you feel your hair starting to stand on end, a lightning strike is imminent. "Get into a catcher's position, crouching on the balls of your feet, lower your head, and cover your ears," says Dr. Cherington. "This is a very bad situation that's best avoided."

Don't go in the water. If you're in your house and the basement has flooded, don't go downstairs to investigate. "You don't know what has happened to the electrical system. The water can be charged and you can get a good shock," Johnson warns. "Once all the water has cleared, don't try restoring the power or heat yourself; you could start a fire. Call professionals."

The Eye of the Storm

When it comes to tropical storms, be thankful that you don't live in Bangladesh. A cyclone on this island south of India wiped out 139,000 people in 1991. Another killed 300,000 in 1970. In other parts of the world, where we give these cyclonic storms pet names and call them hurricanes, the death tolls aren't so dramatic, but the devastation is still enormous. In 1992, Hurricane Andrew killed 14 people and caused an unprecedented billions of dollars in damages. Since then, we're taking hurricanes a little more seriously. You should, too, by heeding these storm warnings.

Shop for the season. If you live in a hurricane-prone area, you should keep your food and medical necessities stocked up during late summer and early fall—prime hurricane season. "After a severe hurricane, you can go as long as seven days without power or transportation," Hudak says.

Listen to the radio. A watch means that a hurricane may hit your area. A warning means that it will. During a watch, make sure that your car has gas; that you have any important papers, IDs, and daily medications that you need; and that you have a well-planned escape route. When there's a warning, bring garbage cans and other large objects inside the garage or house. Shut off water, electricity, and gas. Close your shutters or put up plywood over your windows, says Johnson.

Wait the storm out—completely. If you're there when the storm hits, and you're told not to evacuate, the safest place to be is underground, such as in a basement. Be sure to stay away from windows. Stay tuned to the weather on a battery-powered radio until authorities issue an "all clear," says Johnson. Often when the storm seems to subside, it's really only the calm "eye" of the hurricane and the worst is yet to come. Plus, just to make you feel better, tornadoes can follow hurricanes.

Postwar Trauma

Making It Home

"War is hell."

William Tecumseh Sherman, the Civil War Union general famous for burning Atlanta during his "march to the sea" in 1864, first spoke those infamous words in 1879. Since that day, 618,582 U.S. soldiers have met their maker on the bloody battlefields of war. And that's only half the story. The hell that lives on in the heads of those who make it out of war alive can be comparable to the conflict itself.

In the final analysis, it seems that if you're going to make it through war, you have to survive on two fronts: one, the physical battle of combat itself, and two, battling the memories and mental anguish that follow.

We're not here to tell you how to survive a war if, God forbid, we should have another one. That's a job for the drill sergeants and medics. We're here to give you the experts' advice on how to survive after a war (or for that matter, any long-term life-threatening trauma) and how to live with the memories that can torment for decades after the last bomb has dropped.

System Overload

Even if you've made it home safe and seemingly sound, you may find yourself waging a whole new war— only this time the enemy is you. As one anonymous Vietnam vet puts it, "My marriage is falling apart. . . . I really don't have any friends. . . .

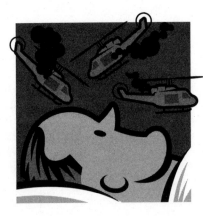

I usually feel depressed. . . . Crowds bother me, so I stay out of malls. And I can't go to the movies either. . . . Loud noises irritate me, and sudden movements or noises make me jump and reach for a weapon. . . . Most of the time I feel like a walking time bomb just looking for a place where I can go off. What the f*** is wrong with me?"

The answer, says Jack Weber, team leader and readjustment counselor at the Vet Center in Evansville, Indiana, is nothing. "That is a perfectly natural response to an absolutely unnatural situation," he says. "It's what we used to call shell shock during World War I and battle fatigue during World War II. Today, we know it as post-traumatic stress disorder (PTSD), and it's a problem that lingers years, often decades, after a soldier comes home.

What happens is that you go through something so horrible and stressful that you disassociate from it, as though it were happening to someone else, says Sylvia Mendel, a trauma consultant in private practice in New York City.

"That's why war victims sound like they're reading from a script when they talk about combat," adds Weber. "Combat also brings your physical stress response to the point of fatigue. You lose your stress response like you would an arm or a leg, and you just can't tolerate stress anymore," Weber says.

As a result, when you return to "normal" conditions, you can't adjust. "Most often, you can no longer get close to people," says Weber. "It's like if you took all of your friends, and each day you lost one. You'd stop having friends. That's what they do."

Veterans often respond suddenly, and often extremely, to what are called triggers—sights, sounds, or smells that remind them of the war. "It could be something obvious like the sound of a plane or a helicopter, or something subtle like the smell of gasoline," says Mendel.

"Sometimes the worst thing is the relentless nightmares," notes Weber.

The Next Wave

Though Vietnam, the war most commonly associated with today's cases of PTSD, was more than 20 years ago, that doesn't mean that you should expect that all these wounds are healed. "You can learn to live with PTSD, but it never fully goes away," says Mendel. In fact, when researchers at the University of Pittsburgh Medical Center surveyed World War II prisoners of war and concentration camp survivors a few years back, they found that about one-third of them still suffered from nightmares and depression more than 45 years later.

What may be more disturbing is that many veterans who seemed to have escaped the worst of PTSD from the Vietnam War are just now beginning to surface with symptoms two decades later. "Many of these men and women came back from the war and completely immersed themselves in their careers, working until they were exhausted every day to numb the pain," says Weber. "But now that they're hitting their fifties, they can't work like they used to and they're losing this coping mechanism. I'm seeing lawyers, physicians, and people from all walks of life who have been extremely functional who are just now breaking down."

The Killing Fields

We've lost enough American soldiers during the past 225 years to populate a small nation. Thankfully, our last battle was our least bloody. The following are principal wars of the United States and how many soldiers we lost on the battlefields alone.

War	Number Serving	Death Count
Revolutionary War (1775–1783)	184,000 to 250,000*	4,435*
War of 1812 (1812–1815)	286,730	2,260*
Mexican War (1846–1848)	78,718	13,283
Civil War (1861–1866)	3,713,363 (estimated Union and Confederate)	498,332
Spanish-American War (1898)	306,760	2,446
World War I (1917–1918)	4,743,826	116,708
World War II (1941–1946)	16,353,659	407,316
Korean War (1950–1953)	5,764,143	33,651*
Vietnam War (1964–1973)	8,744,000	58,168
Persian Gulf War (1991)	467,539	293

*Estimate

Since PTSD increases your risk for suicide, it's important that you seek treatment as soon as you notice symptoms, says Weber. "We can't cure it, but we can make it much easier to live with." Here's what you should know.

Watch the triggers. If you're diving for cover at the sound of a helicopter, that's an obvious sign of PTSD. But some of the things that trigger the onset of the disorder are more subtle, says Mendel. "The losses you experience as you age can bring back all your old unresolved feelings of emotional trauma and trigger PTSD symptoms in the present."

Know your strengths. "Don't for a minute think that you're less of a man if you're having trouble dealing with your trauma," says Weber. "PTSD isn't a weakness; it's a mental condition with physical components. And you owe it to yourself to get help for it."

Walk the wall. A visit to the Vietnam Memorial wall can help, says Weber. "You can go and reconnect with your feelings. You can allow yourself to feel. That's very important for men who have been disconnected from them for so long."

Take yourself in context. "Don't make the mistake of judging what you did in combat by current values," says Weber. "Reframe your actions in the realm of combat. What you did in the context of that situation was okay. You were doing your job."

Find an open ear. You may have felt that you couldn't talk to the people close to you because what you had seen or done seemed too horrible, says Mendel, but there is something very cathartic in finding someone who will listen. "It's best to find someone trained in veteran counseling for that kind of discussion," she notes, "since not just any counselor is prepared to deal with hearing the horrors of combat."

Admit addictions. "Substance abuse and trauma go hand in hand," says Mendel. "If you're using alcohol or drugs to drown your pain, a group like Alcoholics Anonymous can help. But you'll likely also need counseling to deal with the trauma you've been suppressing. The route of relapse in substance abuse is often a trigger of unresolved trauma. This is why counseling on the traumatic events is necessary to avoid relapse."

Hang on. Right now, most therapists use a combination of medications to ease the symptoms of PTSD, says Weber. "But new drugs specific for the condition are being developed as we speak. We should have much better medications in the next few years."

Gradual Decline

We all know how war kills you with a bang. We're now beginning to understand how it kills you with a whisper. PTSD is one way. But researchers from the Carolina Population Center at the University of North Carolina at Chapel Hill also have found that combat veterans from World War II were more likely to experience physical decline and death during the first 15 years after the war than those not involved in combat.

"War is such an incredibly disruptive event," says study author Glen H. Elder Jr., Ph.D., of the Carolina Population Center, "especially when you're mobilized during your late twenties and early thirties like many soldiers were during World War II. This disruption, combined with returning and never really talking about the experience, seems to have had adverse consequences for their physical health, perhaps through an impaired immune function. In our studies, late mobilization and exposure to combat are predictive of declining physical health. There is more cancer and heart disease in the lives of these men."

Echoing those findings, a 50-year study of 152 World War II veterans found that 30 out of 54 veterans who saw intense fighting contracted chronic illnesses and died by the time they were 65. Sixteen of those veterans had complained of symptoms of PTSD. And the rates of disease and death were significantly lower among veterans who had not seen much combat.

Because Vietnam occurred earlier in the soldiers' lives, Dr. Elder isn't able to draw parallels between World War II veterans and those who served in Vietnam. "The disruption occurred when they were younger, but the war had psychological consequences all of its own," he says.

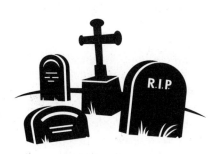

Part Five

Real-Life Scenarios

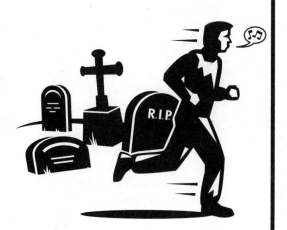

Quest for the Best

These are the champions, my friend. They're at the tops of their fields, despite everything life has thrown at them. They've laughed at death; now they're loving life. And so can you.

You Can Do It!

Time hasn't slowed them down. Disease hasn't stopped them. These guys are living life to the max, and the lessons they've learned are as ageless as they are.

The Quick and the Dead

They were the best at what they did. They had risen to the heights of their professions, earned the respect of their peers. Tragically, their lives were cut short, but we can still learn from how they lived—and how they died.

Quest for the Best
These are the champions, my friend. They're at the tops of their fields, despite everything life has thrown at them. They've laughed at death; now they're loving life. And so can you.

Robert Mondavi, Founder, Robert Mondavi Wineries

Thriving on the Vine of Life

What keeps a man excited about life well into his eighties? A vision. A passion. A joie de vivre. And, in the case of Robert Mondavi, a love of the grape.

"I'm better than ever," immodestly says Mondavi, who was instrumental in helping make wine—and specifically American wine—as popular as it is today. His voice, which booms through the speakerphone from his spacious office at the winery in the heart of Napa Valley, California, carries an almost-palpable vitality.

But even his staff says that sometimes it's hard to keep up with him, despite his age. Mondavi, now in his mid-eighties, explains that his unflagging enthusiasm for life comes from remaining interested in things that are important to him.

Among them are "talking with my grandchildren and educating them about life, so they can live in a permanent state of nirvana," he says. "It's up to them to make life interesting."

A Vision of the Future

His latest passion in promoting wine is helping to make a reality of his dream institute: the American Center for Wine, Food, and the Arts, a center-in-

progress that would continue his efforts to showcase the development of excellent American wines and the culinary, performing, and visual arts. Having a vision is something Mondavi has long been known for. He helped revolutionize the wine industry, convincing consumers that they could have the highest-quality wines at affordable prices. He explains how he rose in his field: "There are many people with vision but few who know how to execute it. There are many intelligent people but not that many with common sense."

Another secret: He knows when to let go. Mondavi has gracefully managed to transfer most of the weighty responsibilities of running the winery to his able sons, Michael (who runs business operations) and Tim (the winemaker). "I am so pleased and proud as a peacock of them," he says. "They're doing a tremendous job. I always thought that, working together, the two of them could do a better job than I ever did. They realize the importance of harmony. They also have vision, and they're learning to delegate authority, supervise properly. Seeing them develop makes *my* life that much more worthwhile."

He also deals with stress differently. "I've

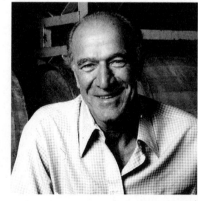

learned after a long time that everyone feels they're right," he says. "At one time I thought I could change people's minds if I used common sense. Then I realized that all of us are different. I can influence someone but not change them. Since I realized getting people to change is no longer my responsibility, I'm a much happier man. I don't get upset. I enjoy life much more than ever before."

Here's another lesson that he has learned that helps him enjoy people a lot more. "The more you give them, the more you get back—if you have patience," he explains.

For the Rest of His Life

In addition, Mondavi has come to terms—reluctantly at first—with the fact that sometimes a man of his age needs a midday rest. And he's not above allowing himself to get pampered a bit. "I've learned that I need rest. I try to get eight hours of rest, but when I don't, I tire out in the middle of the day," he says. "Now I get an hour or two of rest at midday and sometimes a massage, which revives me. With a little rest, I keep going much stronger all day long."

Exercise helps, too, but Mondavi's workout regime is not extraordinary. He does maybe 30 to 40 minutes of exercise: 15 to 20 minutes in a pool, then a walk or jog for another 15 to 20 minutes. The key for him, like the rest of us who are not quite 80 yet, is to do it every day.

Neither is his diet out of the ordinary. "Basically, I've always eaten well—not between meals," he says. In the past several years, he has noticed that he doesn't eat as much as he used to and that he's eating more vegetables, fish, and chicken and less red meat. "But every now and then I love a good steak," he adds. What he now suggests—and the rule he follows—is to eat and drink "in moderation."

As for wine, well, don't get him started. "When I was three or four my mother fed me wine and water, and I've been drinking it since," he says. "Wine was looked upon as a liquid food." He fully supports the research that shows wine, particularly red wine, helps fight heart disease and high cholesterol.

"I am convinced the correlation is there," he says. "I always knew that wine in moderation was good for you. Now there's scientific evidence to prove it. Not only that, but wine is part of culture, part of our heritage and our religion." Mondavi believes that his wine habit is part of the reason for his good health. He drinks two to three glasses of red wine daily.

Naturally, he credits the grape with keeping him hale and hearty and relatively free of illness. Indeed, the only health problem Mondavi has had was back in 1994 when he had surgery for an enlarged prostate. Luckily, there was no cancer involved and he was back at work, at his desk, in the vineyards, traveling the world in less time than you can say Cabernet Sauvignon.

His Cup Runneth Over

There is one other medicinal that has kept Mondavi happy, healthy, and excited about life, especially for the last 17 years. It's love. He was in his late sixties when he married for the second time, to Margrit Biever. "I love her more now than when I married her," he proclaims. "She stimulates me just from the fact that she does so much. She challenges me to keep up with her." Thirteen years his junior, she is a vice president of the winery and actively involved in special events and public relations. She's an excellent cook—the surest way to the heart of an Italian man.

The secret ingredient of their marriage is no secret. "I love her and she loves me," he says succinctly. "We're completely open and honest, and we enjoy being with each other. The only problem is that we're not together enough. Or at least not alone."

For that they plan weekend getaways, for example, up the coast of California to the romantic village of Mendocino. Or they just get in the new Ferrari he bought his wife and drive.

His sheer enjoyment of everything—from his relationship with his wife, to his relationship with his sons and grandchildren, to his ceaseless appreciation of great wine and food, to his passion for a center for food and wine—is almost childlike. And that's just the way he likes it. He is a clear example of a man who, like a good wine, improves with age.

Lance Armstrong, Champion Cyclist

Back in the Saddle Again

Most of us couldn't finish, let alone win, one stage of the grueling 21-day, 3,850-kilometer Tour de France in perfect health.

Now imagine if someone suggested you try doing it with testicular cancer.

Chances are that, even if you were in the shape of your life, you'd figure there was no way you could do it. If you were Lance Armstrong, premier American road cyclist, however, you wouldn't just ride. You'd win. And that's after you had already taken first place in the 12-day, 1,200-mile Tour DuPont for the second year in a row. In 1996, that's exactly what Armstrong did. Only he was so used to riding through pain, he didn't even know he had cancer—until he started coughing up blood, that is.

"I was a pretty sick guy for a long time," recalls Armstrong matter-of-factly. "I had been sore and feeling more fatigued than I should have for the whole season. Nobody knows how long I was racing with cancer, but certainly at least a year, probably longer. At the end, though, I was really sore in my testicles. I also had a severe headache. I had blurry vision. And then I coughed up not just a little but a lot of blood. Obviously, that's not normal. I knew that I couldn't write it off as an athletic injury. I saw a doctor."

That's when the bomb dropped. Right as Armstrong was moving into what could be considered the pinnacle of his cycling career, complete with a Nike endorsement deal and a $2 million contract to compete for France's Team Confidis, he found out that he had testicular cancer. "I simply couldn't believe it. Cancer was the furthest

thing from my mind," recalls Armstrong. Unfortunately, that was just the beginning.

From Bad to Worse

Suspecting that the late-stage testicular cancer had spread, his doctor ordered a chest x-ray. Sure enough, he had cancer there, too. And he had small amounts in his abdominal lymph nodes. Then, several weeks later, Armstrong's news went from really bad to even worse. Further screenings indicated that Armstrong's cancer had also spread to his brain. The 25-year-old was given less than a 50-50 chance to live.

But through it all, Armstrong never said, "Why me?" And he never gave up hope. Instead, he drew on the same strength and perseverance that had propelled him thousands of miles on his bike in all kinds of conditions and across all kinds of terrain. "The way I saw it, my situation was bad, but it wasn't as bad as a lot of other people's. I would look at people who had no hope and put my disease in perspective, just as I hope that people who aren't quite as bad off as I was can look at my situation and gain hope. I was just thankful to have any chance at all."

Over the course of several months, Armstrong underwent extensive chemotherapy, testicular surgery, and then six-hour brain surgery. "That was the worst," he recalls. "Remarkably, though I lost some muscle and gained some fat,

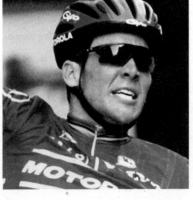

I didn't lose weight during all of it, as sick as I was." Armstrong tips the scales at a solid 170.

Even more remarkably, he got back on his bike just two weeks after each of his surgeries. "Of course, I was just spinning up and down the driveway. I wasn't really riding," he says. But as his treatments continued and his condition improved, Armstrong decided that he really did want to ride again.

In fact, he wanted to race. And with permission from his doctors, "so long as I took it slow," Armstrong started basic training again just 2½ months after being diagnosed with cancer. Then, just one year after he began the biggest battle of—and for—his life, Armstrong made the announcement in 1997 that he had been signed to ride for the U.S. Postal Service Cycling Team, the only American-based cycling team to compete in the Tour de France. It was official; he would race again.

The Ride Back

In the past, Armstrong has been quoted as saying there are two things he likes to do: ride and party. These days he's doing a whole lot of the former and a whole lot less of the latter. He trains seven days a week about four hours a day, working both on the bike and in the weight room. Most nights, he's in bed by 10:00 P.M. Armstrong knows that the next few years are crucial not just for his racing career but for his life.

"No one has ever made a comeback like this before," Armstrong says. "I have enough damage in my body from the cancer that I have to eliminate all the other variables of poor per-formance, whether it's poor training, a bad diet, or lack of motivation. I've always trained hard, but I have never been 100 percent in all those variables. I am now. There are a lot of things that are better now after cancer than they have ever been. My training is better. My fitness level is better. My weight is better."

Plus, cancer is now Armstrong's secret psychological weapon. "Suffering for me is all relative now," he says with a laugh. "If I'm out climbing a big hill on my bike and my heart rate is 190 beats a minute for 10 or 15 minutes, the guy next to me might be thinking, 'Wow, this is terrible.' But I know what terrible really is. That suffering I do on my bike is hardly 1 percent of what I had to go through with cancer. Cancer put everything in perspective.

And I'd much rather be suffering on my bike. That's a big advantage for me now."

The Long Haul

Armstrong wants to help other men beat cancer, too. "So many men will get cancer at some point in their lives. It could be as a young professional athlete or as an old, retired doctor," he says. "We should always be aware of that and not forget to keep a close check on our bodies. If you catch cancer early enough, it's often curable. Too often people don't associate the word *cure* with cancer. But it's true. It can be cured. On the other hand, your cancer won't go away just because you don't know about it. It'll get worse."

It's this kind of advocacy and awareness that Armstrong credits with saving his own life, despite the fact that he admittedly waited much longer than he should have to see a doctor. "If there was no activism on the part of people in the cancer community, I wouldn't be alive today because there never would have been funding for the research. My situation, just 20 short years ago, would have been fatal. We have to get the message out to men to look after their health. And men need to spread the word to others. I'm fortunate that I'm an athlete in a high-profile position. Hopefully, I can reach a lot of people and they'll never have to go through what I did."

Though testicular cancer is rare, it is the most common form of cancer in men ages 20 through 34, with about 7,200 new cases diag-nosed every year. You can help protect yourself by checking your testicles each month (see Medical Testing on page 62). You can also be-come a member of the Lance Armstrong Foun-dation—a nonprofit organization dedicated to raising awareness of urological cancer, raising funds for kids with cancer, and raising money for cancer research. For more information, write to Lance Armstrong Foundation, 111 Congress Avenue, Suite 1400, Austin, TX 78701.

Jack LaLanne, Fitness Icon

On a Mission from God

At age 45, Jack LaLanne completed 1,000 pushups and 1,000 chinups in one hour and 22 minutes. At age 61, he swam the length of the Golden Gate Strait, handcuffed, shackled, and towing a 2,000-pound boat against the tide. At age 70, again handcuffed and shackled, he towed 70 boats with 70 people from Queen's Way Bridge in Long Beach Harbor to the Queen Mary, 1½ miles away. And that's just to name a few famous feats.

Is he mad? Perhaps. But more than that, LaLanne has a higher purpose. "I take my lead from Jesus," says LaLanne. "Not that I would *ever* compare myself to Him, but Jesus performed wonderful miracles to call attention to His message. I wanted to do that, too."

Now in his mid-eighties, he still does. LaLanne admits that some folks find him a tad fanatical. But what they don't understand is that he's a man with a mission. And he's not leaving this earth until he's through. "I haven't done a thing yet," says LaLanne when you mention his many amazing accomplishments. "I can't think about dying. I have so much to do. And though my message is more accepted today than it used to be, there are millions of people whom I still need to reach."

Believe, Believe

It's hard to believe, now that everyone and his grandmother is hoisting free weights, but in the 1930s when LaLanne first started making a name for himself as a paragon of health and fitness, he had more than his share of doubting Thomases trying to run him out of town.

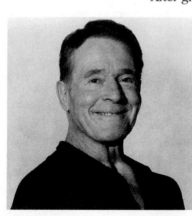

One reason was that when LaLanne first started preaching the benefits of nutrition and exercise, he was practically all alone. It started when he was 15. With his father already dead by his midforties from "unhealthy living," LaLanne was, by his own admission, one sickly adolescent. "I was 30 pounds underweight. I lived off junk food. I had pimples, boils, glasses, arch supports, and one sickness after another," recalls LaLanne. Things got so bad, he left school for six months due to ill health and began a downward spiral. "I was thinking about suicide. It just seemed hopeless. Then our next-door neighbor Mrs. Joy told my mother to take me to hear a health lecture by this man named Paul Bragg. He saved my life that night," says LaLanne. "He said that it didn't matter what condition you were in or how old you were. If you followed nature's laws, you could be reborn. And man, did I want to be reborn."

LaLanne wasted no time. "I gave up white flour and white sugar. I joined the local YMCA. I became a vegetarian. And I bought *Gray's Anatomy* and read it cover to cover. I started working out and became captain of the football team and state wrestling champion. Then, in 1931, while I was still at Berkeley, California, High School, I bought dumbbells and opened my first gym in my backyard. I would train local police officers and firemen and sell seeds, dates, honey, and other health foods. My fellow students shunned me. Lots of people thought I was nuts," he says. And that was before he went public.

After graduating from chiropractic college, LaLanne opened his first real gym, complete with carpeted floors and mirrored walls. At a time when gyms were dark, dank places called sweat boxes, where only boxers went, no one had ever seen anything like it. "Doctors would actually tell their patients not to see me because I was a 'dumb nut,' a 'cheat' and a 'crook,'" LaLanne laughs. "They would tell women not to lift weights because they'd look like men. They would actually tell athletes not to lift weights because they would get so muscle-bound that they wouldn't be able to perform. That's when I started doing all those swimming events to show them they were wrong."

Thirty-four years of syndicated workout shows and a half-dozen books later, LaLanne has been vindicated. In fact, there's talk of LaLanne putting together a new television show, once again showing millions of Americans the benefits of nutrition and exercise.

Built with Pride

Sure, you say. It's easy for Jack LaLanne to swim lots of miles, lift lots of weights, and keep in shape. That's what he gets paid for. But LaLanne begs to differ. "C'mon, guys. Be honest with yourselves. How many hours do you waste watching TV? Yeah, if you want to perform amazing feats, you have to work out more. But for the average person, investing a half-hour to an hour, three or four times a week, is plenty."

Good health, no matter what your age, simply takes pride and discipline, says LaLanne. "You think I like to leave a hot woman and a warm bed to get up at 5:00 A.M. and go to a cold gym? Absolutely not. But I love the results. We all hate to train. But it doesn't take much to reap huge benefits. Get up. Stretch. Do some pushups. Go for a vigorous walk. Live with enthusiasm and energy. Don't be like so many millions of Americans and start dying from your own bad habits and lack of enthusiasm as soon as you hit 30. Your body is the only machine that gets better the more you use it."

Besides hard work and discipline, what has kept Jack LaLanne's biceps bulging against his Lycra sleeves all these decades? "I keep aiming higher," he says. Here are a few tips on how the quintessential Mr. America got and stayed where he is today.

• No rest. "I see these guys waiting minutes between sets at the gym. You should lift to fatigue and rest only 10 seconds between sets for maximum strength and endurance," he says.

• Write it down and shake it up. "Write down exactly what you're doing. Do it for three weeks. Then change it," advises LaLanne. "If you've been lifting low weight at high repetitions, start lifting more weight fewer times. Do that for three weeks, and change again. That keeps your muscles developing and your mind from getting bored."

• Pop those pills. No matter how good your diet, you should consider vitamin and mineral supplements to put back what is taken from your food during processing and cooking, says LaLanne.

• Push the envelope. Complacency is your enemy. Always strive for a higher goal and a new challenge. "I'd swim from Alcatraz to San Francisco in handcuffs one year. Then the next year I'd do it again, only I'd pull a boat, too. Now that people are saying I'm too old for those stunts, I'd like to swim the 26 miles from Catalina Island to Los Angeles underwater—with oxygen provided from a boat above. You just can't stop."

Well, let him amend that. If you're going to stop anything, stop filling your body with junk, pleads LaLanne. "Society has gone so far awry with its eating habits. Turn on your television right now and all you'll see are advertisements telling you to drink sugar-filled soft drinks and eat foods loaded with butter, cream, and cheese. That's not to mention all the magazines telling you to smoke cigarettes and drink booze. People get addicted to all of these things. And they drag the country down, leaving millions of people feeling lousy."

In the final analysis, that's why LaLanne believes he's here: to help us save ourselves. "I can't leave this planet yet. There are millions of people out there drowning in that lake of bad health and lack of enthusiasm. They're going down for the third time, and I have to reach out my hand and pull them in. The biggest measure of the quality and success in life is how many people you can help. And I have a lot yet to do."

Gregory White Smith, Pulitzer Prize– Winning Author

Making a Miracle

Gregory White Smith was 34 when neurosurgeons at the prestigious Mayo Clinic in Rochester, Minnesota, told him his number was up. A benign growth in his head had turned suddenly and unexpectedly malignant, leaving the New York City author facing an inoperable brain tumor. His doctors gave him "three months, maybe six" to live.

That was more than 10 years ago.

Today, Smith is still around to tell his story. And he has not merely survived; he has thrived. He went on to write a Pulitzer Prize–winning biography of artist Jackson Pollock and, most recently, a book about his long medical battle. It's called, aptly enough, *Making Miracles Happen.*

Smith's diagnosis came a few days before Christmas 1986, and he needed a miracle. Smith had traveled unaccompanied to snowy Minnesota for his exam and left the doctor's office feeling more alone than ever before. The cold news contrasted starkly with the cheery carols echoing through the hospital halls. "The seasonal gaiety made the bleak news seem even more surreal, harder to absorb. The fact that it came from such a reputable institution made it even harder to deny," Smith writes.

On his own in a strange town, with time to ponder an untimely death, Smith's first response was to gorge on comfort food. "I went back to my hotel and ate every cinnamon bun in the coffee shop," he recalls.

But later that day in his hotel room, Smith also had a realization that would literally save his life. While watching a dismal television weather forecast, he saw a correlation between the weather report and his doctor's diagnosis.

Much like meteorologists making forecasts based on past weather patterns, Smith's physicians were only making predictions based on past experience with similar patients. "They were using a statistical table," Smith realized, "not a crystal ball.

"What they really meant was not that I would die in three months but that a substantial majority of patients with symptoms like mine died within three months," recalls Smith. "A substantial majority, but not all. All I had to do was figure out how to beat the odds."

Whose Life Is It?

What does it feel like to be told you have a terminal illness? It's a frantic, silent helplessness, a sense of disconnection from the world and everything familiar and secure, says Smith. It is a sense of isolation and a speeding of time when you desperately want it to slow down. Perhaps what hit Smith hardest of all, though, was the feeling that he had suddenly lost control of his life. This was not a feeling he was accustomed to.

"Suddenly, the one thing you thought you had complete dominion over, your body, is in open revolt; and the one thing most important to you, your future, is in somebody else's hands. No wonder people suddenly see their

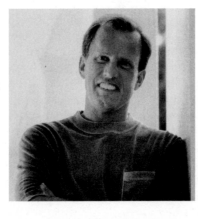

lives as well as their bodies spinning out of control," says Smith.

So Smith tried to get back some of that control. He went for a second opinion. Was the tumor operable? Would radiation help? But the answers were the same: No. "That stopped me," says Smith. "Going to a third doctor to hear the same thing was unthinkable." To him, a second opinion was nothing more than a confirmation and a reassurance that the last word was really the last word. And for his case, the last word was clearly a negative one. He would soon find that to be untrue.

"No one has the last word, except you," Smith recalls being told by actor Charles Grodin when they met at a party. Grodin's ex-wife had just died of cancer, and he knew what he was talking about. "There's a whole world of experimental protocols out there, people pursuing unusual things, people who aren't happy with conservative answers, people looking for other answers," writes Smith of Grodin's advice. "You haven't even begun to fight." Smith realized that he was right. Seeing two doctors and quitting was ridiculous. Smith decided that the only way to take back control of his life was to take control of his illness.

Taking Charge Again

"I decided that there must be options, and my job was to find them," says Smith. He decided that he would go anywhere, talk to anyone, read anything, follow any lead, turn any stone. He boned up on the most cutting-edge research and sought out experimental treatments so new that they hadn't even been published.

"I hunted down every piece of information on my condition that I could find and discovered a doctor who didn't think I was a lost cause," Smith recalls. Working with that doctor, Smith was able to try an experimental hormone therapy that stopped the cancer from growing. He had made the miracle happen.

And that's what he recommends to others who face similar battles: "The best strategy for a man who wants to live," suggests Smith, is to "scour the Internet to find abstracts, the library to find articles, periodicals . . . you name it. But you must realize that everything published is about three to five years behind the cutting edge of research. To find truly up-to-the-minute information, you have to track down the doctors who are actually conducting the studies. These people not only know the latest research but,

even more important, also can speculate about where that research is leading. They can take you out beyond the cutting edge. You won't get that from your local hospital, and it may be the very information you need to survive."

Smith's message—and the message of *Making Miracles Happen*—is not just one of control of your illness and your life but also one of hope. "Regardless of what any physician might tell you, there are very few problems that don't have at least two possible treatments," Smith says. "The purpose of doing all this research is to come up with these options. Some treatments may be experimental, but doctors from reputable institutions are conducting trials all over the world. Find one and beg or borrow to get in."

To avoid "chasing rainbows," however, make sure that every doctor you speak with is as good as or better than the last one. "If you start with physicians at well-known institutions, who've published research, then work your way up, you won't wind up being treated at Joe's Bait Shop and Cancer Clinic," he says.

How do you make a medical miracle happen? Control, hope, and support are the key ingredients. "Take away a patient's sense of control over his life and you have hurt him more than any injury or disease," says Smith. "Give him back that sense of control and you have helped him more than any drug or therapy."

As for hope, Smith says that there are medical technologies being seen today that would have been indistinguishable from a miracle as recently as 5 to 10 years ago. As long as you stick with legitimate treatment, you can never look too hard to find the right options for yourself. "The only false hope is uninformed hope," says Smith.

But support is what makes the real difference. It is "the final ingredient—after the right doctor, the right treatment, and the right attitude—for making medical miracles happen," he says. "Support can instill the will to live where it doesn't exist, or strengthen it where it does." In the end, it may be the greatest miracle of all.

You Can Do It! Time hasn't slowed them down. Disease hasn't stopped them. These guys are living life to the max, and the lessons they've learned are as ageless as they are.

A Century of Progress

Harry Foesig,
Lansdale, Pennsylvania

Date of birth: August 7, 1897

Profession: Retired engineer and artist

I've been asked a million times, and my answer is always the same: There isn't any secret regimen or magic diet responsible for my 100-plus years of living. But maybe it's the way I've always looked at life that has helped me live it for so long.

You don't get to be my age and not see a lot of history unfold before your eyes. I've lived through the Great Depression, Prohibition, and every major world war. I can remember when a tub of water and a washboard were the only way to wash your clothing, and when automobiles, telephones, and running water were rare luxuries.

My earliest memory dates back to 1900, riding a brand-new tricycle that my uncle gave me as a birthday gift. I remember repeatedly riding that tricycle over bumps near the storefronts of the neighborhood in which I lived. It's strange, the things you so vividly remember.

I've lived in the Philadelphia area my entire life, and I've had quite a varied career. I graduated high school in 1915 and then took classes in engineering and industrial arts at local colleges. I even received a full scholarship to attend the University of Pennsylvania, but because education wasn't as valued as it is today, my parents encouraged me to take more "practical" courses at another nearby school. I started working as a structural engineer, but after losing my job during the Depression, I had to fall back upon my artistic talent. That "practical" art training came in handy, as I was able to support myself during these lean years as a freelance commercial artist. Then with the coming of World War II, I was able to find work as a draftsman.

The happiest moment of my life was marrying my wife, Martha, in 1924. We've been married for 74 years and have 2 children, 6 grandchildren, 22 great-grandchildren, and 2 great-great-grandchildren. Martha began receiving personal care several years ago, so she moved to the retirement home in which we currently live. Because of the special care she requires, we live on different floors. But I spend as much time with her as I possibly can. Like any other, our marriage has had its rough spots, but Martha has been the most wonderful wife. Her love and support have enabled me to achieve all that I have.

Taking It Easy, Keeping It Active

If I had to assign a common theme to my life, it would be moderation. I remember when alcohol was completely outlawed in the 1920s during Prohibition. But, to the surprise of many people today, Prohibition didn't really affect me—as I've always lived my life in moderation. Similarly, I've always been a mild-mannered person. I don't let people upset me, nor do I lose my temper easily. If I became upset each time life threw a curve ball, I might not have made it to 100. Living life one day at a time has more or less been my mantra.

My life has been filled with a plethora of interests and activities, and I've always been active in my community. I've been a town councilman, building inspector, and president of the local library board. And back in 1964 I managed to put my engineering and building skills to use when I built an entire house for my mother.

I truly believe that you can't have too many interests in life. Trolley cars and baseball have been longtime hobbies of mine. In fact, I've had such an interest in trolley cars that I've had three books published on them.

I've even serendipitously stumbled upon a few hobbies. When my wife broke a leg some years back and wasn't able to maneuver around the kitchen, I was forced to learn how to cook. This opened up a whole new world for me, and now I enjoy cooking immensely. Making soup (I can cook up more than 10 varieties) is my specialty.

I know it's the hobby of many, but I don't quite understand the ongoing obsession that society has with television. I've always regarded sitting idly in front of the television as a large waste of time, and I think it prevents people from really living their life. But I do enjoy watching the news and an occasional baseball game.

Age Adjustments

I retired in 1962, but like many others, I found retirement life to be a bit dull. In an effort to remain active, I started writing a weekly column and drawing cartoons on politics and goings-on for the local newspaper. I continued to write during my retirement for almost 20 years. Writing this column helped me to stay involved and active in the community; it gave me a weekly challenge.

Of course, things in your life change when you reach my age. I was able to drive until I was 96, and I would frequently go to area baseball games. But now that I can't drive,

I've lost a good portion of my independence. I am fortunate that I have a daughter and son who frequently visit me and take me shopping and to appointments. I'm not as active as I once was, but I try to keep my time occupied by visiting my wife and daughter and doing cryptograms and playing solitaire. I also take naps during the day. At my age, I figure I'm entitled to it.

It's difficult not to get the blues when you realize that almost everyone you knew when you were young is no longer living. But visits from my grandchildren always help to counter these feelings.

Another thing that has helped me keep a good attitude about life is my health. Believe it or not, I've never been seriously ill, and I can't recall that I've even ever had a headache. I continue to feel unusually healthy, and I don't have any serious medical conditions. I do have some of the common conditions associated with old age: I started to lose my hearing about 10 years ago, and I also have a touch of arthritis. I use a walker to get around as my legs are a little wobbly, but I can walk without it. And I still have a full head of hair—not even a bald spot.

Luck has also played a part in my longevity. I don't think I could have done it without the superior longevity genes I inherited from my parents. As far as I know, I come from a long line of nonagenarians. I also had a cousin who lived to 107.

Living my life in moderation and keeping active in mind and body has helped me make it to the major leagues of life. But, most important, I've been able to surround myself and my life with caring family and friends and a loving and supportive wife. All of these factors have enabled me to live a full life, and I'm too stubborn to stop now. The current world record for the oldest person was held by that 122-year-old French woman. I received three birthday parties when I turned 100; I can only imagine the parties when I break this record.

Running for His Life

Bob Littky,
Farmington Hills, Michigan

Date of birth: March 22, 1935

Profession: Retired printer

I'm 63 years old, and my doctor tells me that I have the body of a 40-year-old man. And that's after having a heart attack, triple bypass surgery, and a stroke.

How did I go from staring death in the face to staring at Mr. Fit in the mirror? I just put one foot in front of the other.

At age 48 I was 50 pounds overweight and smoked three packs of cigarettes a day. I wasn't exercising and was exhausted most of the time. I ran the printing business my father had started nearly 50 years before. Now I was the owner, and I was under a lot of pressure. I would get up at 2:00 in the morning, light a cigarette, and do some more work. I just had so much on my mind. I said to my wife, "If this doesn't get better, I'm going to have a heart attack."

One morning, that's exactly what happened. I woke up with this tingling sensation on my left side that went all the way down to my hand. It didn't hurt; it just felt funny. I went to work and afterward my wife, Loretta, and I went out to dinner. When we got home from the restaurant, I said to her, "Honey, I think I have a problem. It's been bothering me all day." We called 911, and they took me to the hospital.

The doctor said that it was a good thing I got checked out. He said the tingling would go away in a few hours and I would think everything was fine. But everything was not fine; the doctor said that I had suffered a minor heart attack the day before. He said these heart attacks often go unnoticed, and then two or three years later you suffer another more severe heart attack that usually lands you in a wooden box

surrounded by flowers, rather than just laying you up in the hospital for a few days.

I was lucky, in a way. Not only did I have a minor heart attack but also the doctor soon discovered that my arteries were blocked. He said that I could either have triple bypass surgery or spend the rest of my life sitting around, unable to work. Two more doctors checked out my ticker and said the same thing. Loretta wasn't sure if I should have the surgery, but I said, "Let's do it. We'll do a bypass, and I'll change my lifestyle." And I did.

On the Road to Recovery

After the surgery, my doctor had me on more medications than a pharmacist fills in a day. I wanted to try and get off the meds if I could, so I went to see another doctor. This guy told me that if I changed my diet, lost some weight, and exercised, I might be able to stop taking the pile of pills. "Let's try it for six months and see if it works," he said.

I started running with a few other heart patients as part of the hospital's rehabilitation program. Once we were in better shape, the seven of us started racing—and I loved it. Then I heard about a man who had walked and jogged a marathon after having a heart attack. "*I* want to do that," I said. So I went to my doctor (who happened to be a runner himself) and asked if I could run a marathon. He said, "Sure, as long as you train properly."

After six months, I had lost 50 pounds and had begun training for my first marathon. I also made a lot of changes to my diet. At the advice of my doctor, I was eating chicken, turkey, fish, pasta, and lots of vegetables. No red meat, dairy products, or eggs. Before the heart attack, I ate meat and potatoes, meat and potatoes, meat and potatoes. Pizza had been a staple food for me. And I couldn't remember when a vegetable had last shown up on my plate.

Believe it or not, it really wasn't that difficult to change how I ate. The people at the hospital taught my wife how to cook the stuff so that it would be healthy but still taste good. I have to admit that I wasn't crazy about eating fish. As a kid, I remember when my mother would make fish—the whole house would smell of Charlie the Tuna. But I tried all kinds of fish cooked a bunch of different ways, and I found some that I really like.

A Stroke of Bad Luck

A year after my heart attack, I was lean and limber and ready to run my first marathon. Three days before the race, I was out for a run and I got this horrible headache. So I ran home and went to sleep. When Loretta came home, she found me in a coma. They rushed me to the hospital, where one doctor said I was a goner. But another doctor said that he would try to save me, if he could.

He did brain surgery to clip a ruptured aneurysm, which is a blood vessel that had burst in my brain. Two days later, a second blood vessel burst in my brain and he had to operate again. The doctor said that the aneurysms had caused a stroke, which means that part of my brain was damaged. He said that I was born with the two weakened blood vessels and they just gave out.

I don't remember everything that happened after the stroke, but my wife and four kids do. They tell me that I was in the hospital for a month. I remember that the television would be on, but I didn't understand what the people on TV were talking about. I also remember being extremely hungry. I was on these steroid drugs the doctors gave me, and they made me hungry all of the time. Sometimes I would be walking and I would suddenly fall down. I recognized my family, but I couldn't always say their names. I would know what I wanted to say, but my mouth wouldn't say the words. Reading was really difficult. I still have trouble reading sometimes. And numbers were tough. I couldn't add or tell time—and I

had been an accountant before joining my father's printing business. I had lost some of my peripheral vision, so I couldn't drive. And I certainly couldn't go back to work. I knew I had a long road ahead of me.

Back on Track

When I left the hospital, I wanted to start running again. About a month after my stroke, I went for a short run. And after a quarter of a mile, I suddenly didn't know where I was. It was scary. But I didn't let that fear keep me from running. Soon I was training for another marathon. My doctors were a bit concerned because they weren't completely certain what was going on in my brain. So when I ran my first marathon on October 13, 1985, they ran it with me. They wanted to make sure that I knew where I was at all times. Five doctors ran by my side in Detroit. One ran the first mile, another ran the next five miles, and so on. I finished in 5:26:20.

Since then I've run 16 more marathons, including two Bostons and one 3:30 marathon in Detroit. I run 50 races a year, and one or two of those are marathons. I love the action. I never sit. I'm at the health club at the crack of dawn, lifting weights or doing the rowing machine. Fifteen years ago I would eat and smoke while I watched TV. Now I'm on the treadmill. I like to bike, too. Every day I run and jog with each of my four dogs. I exercise between one and three hours a day, even more if I'm training for a marathon. I take vitamins and herbs, and the only medication I take is baby aspirin. I have so much energy now that it makes people nervous.

This is how I want to live. I may have run 17 marathons, but I'm not ready to hang up my running shoes just yet. I've looked death in the face twice and have come away the winner. As far as life's finish line goes, I'm still miles and miles away from reaching the end of this race.

The Will to Live

James Pfister,
Carmi, Illinois

Date of birth: June 16, 1948

Profession: Veterans representative

I'll tell you one thing. There's nothing in life that is too rough to handle. Nothing. You can take the biggest mess, and you can either live in that mess or decide to chip away at it until there is no mess anymore. It's all about making decisions.

I joined the Army when I was 17. I volunteered for Vietnam when I was 18, and away I went in November 1966. In the beginning, I was a clerk, but I didn't feel like I was doing much to help the war effort. So I extended my tour of duty six months and became a helicopter door gunner. In January 1968, we got shot down and captured. I ended up spending the next five years in captivity as a prisoner of war, until they signed the peace agreements out of Paris in 1973 and we were finally sent home.

That one experience changed everything. It was like the whole rug had been pulled out from beneath my feet, and I was left there saying, "What happened?" I had to reconstruct my whole self. My way of thinking, my disposition, my roots, even my metabolism— everything had to change. I had to ask myself, Do I want to take the easy way out and just let myself die here and get it over with? Or do I want to stick this thing out and live? I did not want to die and be buried in Vietnam, so I figured, "I can do this."

Only the Strong Survive

In the end, hard times teach you an awful lot about yourself. I remember being in that prisoner-of-war camp, and they were telling us we had to carry 18-foot-long logs a mile from the field back to the camp so that we could chop them up and cook our own rice. I thought, "You have got to be joking me." I had lost 30 pounds. I had been through dysentery, malaria, beriberi, jungle rot, and general malnutrition, and there I was doing manual labor. I said, "God, Pfister, I didn't know you could do this!" Heck, I didn't even have a big red "S" on my chest. It was then that I learned what I was capable of doing.

The toughest part really was right in the beginning. After the first eight months, I was really homesick. I missed the United States. I didn't know how on earth I was going to survive. I just stopped eating, and I got pretty sick. That's when a buddy of mine said, "You better snap out of this because once you're too far gone, that's it. You end up dying." That's when I got my head out of the old echo chamber, got up on my feet, and got active.

For the first three years of captivity, we were in the jungles of South Vietnam. So food was very hard to come by. All we got was that one bowl of rice each day. So I would use the rice to lure chickens into camp. When I couldn't get a chicken, I would eat snakes, toads, frogs, lizards, even rats. Anything for a meat ration. I'd always share, though not many people took me up on the rat. For vegetables, we'd pull weeds, boil them, and eat them. If we didn't get sick, we'd eat them again the next day. We learned how to get by as well as we could. And it paid off. I ended up being one of the five strong people in our camp who helped those who were less fortunate.

After two years, I figured we were going to be there for the duration. Then at the end of that year, they hiked us up to North Vietnam. We walked the whole way. It took 45 days. And after two years there, we got the word that we would finally be going home. I just couldn't believe it until our aircraft was off the ground.

We had been imprisoned for 5 years and 2 months. I had been in Vietnam for 6½ years total.

Perseverance Pays Off

When I got back, they offered me a state job in Indiana. But I figured the best thing for me would be to re-enlist in the military. I finished out my military career in Fort Bliss, Texas. And after I had my 20 years in, which included Vietnam, I retired. Here I was, 38 years old, and I was like a lost kid, with no idea how to survive in the civilian world.

I applied for Veterans Administration disability in 1986 and found out that I had post-traumatic stress disorder. I guess I knew I had a problem but never gave it a name. I had nightmares five to seven times a week that would make me scream bloody murder in the middle of the night. I still do. But at least now I've come to terms with my situation and my disabilities. But it was a struggle for a while. I had a very short fuse and wasn't able to get close to people. I ended up going through 13 or 14 jobs. I also had a couple of failed marriages. I just moved from state to state. I don't even know what I was looking for.

Finally, I applied for a state job in Evansville, Indiana. Thirteen months later, they called me for an interview; four days later, I got the job as a veterans representative. Now, I talk with veterans and try to help them with job placement and job training. I also try to talk to them about their losses and their problems so that I can point them in the right direction for help. I've already been there; I've done it. Now I'm a stepping-stone for these men. I care. I will listen. Many of these men have no idea about the benefits they're entitled to, especially if they have post-traumatic stress disorder. It's very rewarding to help them. I also try to help kids when I can. I speak to the kids at the local high schools about making decisions in life. They're the people who are going to take my place someday. And I hope they can learn from my experience as well.

Life Is Good

I have never looked back and regretted. I made the decision to be a helicopter door gunner. And, well, sometimes stuff happens. I don't blame myself for it. The way we were shot down, with both of our hydraulic modules being knocked out, was a one-in-a-million shot. But sometimes you're a statistic. I am not going to dote on the bad things that have happened in my life. I am not going to pout about past history. I served my country very honorably. I proved to myself what I am capable of doing when push comes to shove.

And while I can't do much now because I have spinal arthritis in my back (from an injury I got in the helicopter crash), I can still do a lot more than a lot of other men who were hurt worse than I was. I do what I can do. And if I can't do everything that I'd like to, I don't let it put me on my behind. I can still go outside and garden. I can still fish in the spring and the summer. I can still do a good bit of yard work. And all that is better than sitting inside feeling sorry for myself and doing nothing at all.

I have a good outlook on life, and I have a wife whom I would die for. She understands me and is there for me. My life is a comfortable one, and my work helping veterans is very rewarding. I feel as if the tribulations I've experienced were part of life's master plan, and this plan brought me to the place I am today. My experience in Vietnam was a part of my life that is now a part of me. Maybe I wouldn't be the person I am now, had I not experienced all that I have. We truly are the sum of our experiences.

Marathon Man

Bill Brobston,
DeLand, Florida

Date of Birth: January 11, 1913

Profession: Retired president, Alpha Portland Cement

Most people think it's a little unusual that I run marathons, especially since I didn't start running at all until I was 58. And that was about 30 years ago.

A lot of men live into their late eighties, but how many make it that far and can say that they feel healthier than when they were 40? I can, and I owe it to running and my other favorite exercises. And I know that if I continue to exercise, I'll keep living life to its fullest in the years to come.

Though running is my favorite form of exercise, I try to vary my activities. My wife, Erlinda, and I start each day with a brisk walk as the sun's coming up. After breakfast, three days a week Erlinda and I play mixed doubles tennis with another couple. If it isn't a tennis morning, I drag my dog, Red, out for a six- to eight-mile run on one of the local trails. My afternoon is usually devoted to our garden—Erlinda and I are avid gardeners. And I try to get away to the mountains to hike and camp whenever I can (though I don't camp too often anymore now that I'm getting up there in years).

A Late Start

I haven't always been this active. Of course, I played sports when I was younger—football, baseball, and downhill skiing while I was in college. I even played the tennis tournament circuit for a short while after college. But once I started working and I had a family to support, I didn't make the time for good habits. I had four children to raise and a job in sales that didn't leave me with a lot of time for leisure

activities. It also didn't help that one of the perks of being a salesman was a big expense account. Buying drinks and dinner for clients regularly was an easy way to get offtrack when it came to my health.

I got back into exercise at the ripe age of 58 because of an illness, but it was my son's, not mine. My youngest son, Bill Jr., was stricken with scoliosis, a curvature of the spine. His doctor suggested that he take up running to strengthen his back and inhibit the curvature. We weren't getting along so well at the time—you know how fathers and sons sometimes are. But I knew that he wouldn't stick with a running program on his own, so I agreed to run with him. This ailment of my son's changed my life. It reformed me from a 195-pound heavy smoker and drinker into a 145-pound runner. I've been running ever since. And beyond all the great health benefits regular exercise has given me, it helped settle whatever disagreements my son and I had. All those miles on the road together gave us an opportunity to be great friends, and we still are today.

Breaking Records

I've come a long way since my first couple of laps around the block almost 30 years ago. It has been a struggle, but I continued to train. I've been fortunate that no injuries or health problems have disrupted my exercise schedule. In fact, running probably helped save my health.

And for those days that are really tough, I've learned some tricks that keep me from shortening my practice runs. I'll have my wife drop me off six miles from home, and then I have no choice but to run every inch of the way back.

I now run in races on a regular basis, and I run at least one marathon every year just to keep in shape. I've run the New York City Marathon, Boston Marathon, and the Marine Corps Marathon in Washington, D.C. Right now

I am training for the National Marathon Masters Championship in Minneapolis/St. Paul. I'm very excited for this year's marathon because now I'm in a new age bracket—the 85-to-89 age group. For the moment, I'll be the "kid" in the group. My goal is to establish a record for this age bracket, just as I did when I entered a new age group at 80.

Even though I started exercising later than others, I've won a lot of awards as a golden-ager both in running and tennis. I hold a record in the half-marathon for runners over 70 with a time of 1:36—that works out to just under 8-minute miles. My personal record for a marathon is 3:33—just over 8-minute miles. I've been named Runner of the Year by the New York Road Runners Club. And just before I left Saugerties, New York, to move to a warmer climate (that huge snowstorm in 1993 had me packing my bags for Florida), I won the New York seniors doubles tennis championship.

But probably the accomplishment I am most proud of is my 6½-day, 145-mile run from Saugerties to Easton, Pennsylvania. That breaks down to a marathon a day, for six concurrent days. I'm a history buff, and this run was a journey for me down the Old Mine Road—the route that was used during the Revolutionary times to haul iron from the Catskills to New Jersey. Though this was an exciting run for me, I did it more for the community than for myself. I used this run as a way to raise money for an academic scholarship to the community college in Saugerties. People pledged money for each mile that I ran. It was quite a successful run for me, and Saugerties Community College. The school now has a scholarship in my name.

Being involved in the community is very important to me. I like to use my good health and love of running to do good for others. It helps me set new goals that get me out and running on those days that I just want to curl up with a good book. It's tough to train when you're in your late eighties; it's tough to train at any age. But I enjoy competition, and I love

winning. And all this exercise and running keeps me on a perpetual runner's high.

A Strong Finish

I'm also a great believer in eating well. Before I started exercising, I wasn't very careful about my diet. But once I started walking, running, and playing tennis, that had to change. I had to be well-fueled so that I could keep up with my son on the streets and my wife on the courts. Now I watch my diet—well, my wife watches it for me. Instead of martinis, I now drink orange juice. And I eat plenty of healthy foods like whole grains, fruits, vegetables, nuts, and legumes.

My wife and I share a pretty good life together. Besides our physical activities, we read and write regularly to keep our minds sharp, and we get plenty of rest so that we're fresh each day. Erlinda and I have a great relationship. We take care of each other. It's a good trade-off. She's my loudest cheerleader at races, and my support crew on longer runs. Both of us have a real passion for life and each other. If the passion were gone between us, Erlinda would divorce me.

I truly believe that everything happens for the best. If it hadn't been for my son's unfortunate/fortunate ailment, I probably would be dead. I'm not quite the last leaf on the tree, but most of my generation has pretty well passed along. The fact that I love athletics keeps me around and running. (I think I also got lucky with some long-living genes in my family.)

It helps that I'm a positive thinker with high energy. The old expression that "growing older is a state of mind" is very true. You need a young, positive outlook on life, and you can't really have one unless your health is good. Since I have been taking care of my health, I find that a lot of the other problems I had seem to take care of themselves. The benefits of being health-conscious are far too great to stop now.

The Quick and the Dead

They were the best at what they did. They had risen to the heights of their professions, earned the respect of their peers. Tragically, their lives were cut short, but we can still learn from how they lived—and how they died.

William Henry Harrison

Long-Winded and Short-Lived

The 1840 U.S. presidential election was the first truly modern political campaign. William Henry Harrison, as the Whig candidate, and his supporters blanketed the country with appearances and speeches on the candidate's behalf. It was a "long, very, very windy" campaign, says William Shade, Ph.D., professor of history at Lehigh University in Bethlehem, Pennsylvania.

After winning the hard-fought election, Harrison headed straight for Washington to begin a dizzying round of meetings. It was the first time the Whigs, a new political party, were in office. He had to meet with the heads of his party and others who had helped him during the election. A Cabinet also had to be selected.

The popular belief was, and continues to be, that Harrison's busy schedule, coupled with his advanced age of 68 (very old, at a time when the average American man lived to be 47), and his inability to slow down, broke down his body's resistance. Then he capped it off by giving the longest inaugural address on record—1 hour and 40 minutes—outdoors, on a freezing March day, without wearing a coat or hat. President Harrison followed that up by partying at numerous inaugural balls throughout the night. Many people thought his body thanked him by catching a cold—a cold that developed into pneumonia.

The physicians who attended the ailing president described his condition on March 27 as "bilious pleurisy, with symptoms of pneumonia and intestinal inflammation," which sounds pretty bad by the standards of any century. Harrison died on April 4, 1841, one month to the day after delivering his chilly inaugural address.

Did a cold coupled with exhaustion cause Harrison's pneumonia and eventually his death? According to Steven Mostow, M.D., professor of medicine at the University of Colorado in Denver and chairman of the American Thoracic Society's Committee on the Prevention of Pneumonia and Influenza, in New York City, the answer is no. What probably caused Harrison's death wasn't a cold but a mild to moderate case of influenza that eventually developed into pneumonia. Dr. Mostow says that the cold virus doesn't attack the lining of the lung; it attacks only the lining of the nose and throat. "He probably caught influenza from someone he shook hands with or who sneezed on him, and that became bacterial pneumonia,"

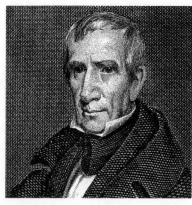

Dr. Mostow says. "Today, he could have prevented this by getting a flu shot." Modern medicine also offers a pneumonia vaccine, he adds.

Still, Harrison could have taken better care of himself. While the long-winded speech itself didn't cause Harrison's pneumonia, he certainly wasn't doing his 68-year-old body any favors by exposing it to harsh cold on that fateful day.

Mickey Mantle

How the Mick Struck Out

Nobody could make a bat crack like Mickey Mantle did. As soon as you heard that distinctive sound, you knew that it was going out of the park. Raised in the poor mining town of Spavinaw, Oklahoma, Mickey Charles Mantle had joined the New York Yankees in 1951 at age 19 and eventually became the worthy successor to the great center fielder Joe DiMaggio. Mantle's powerful switch-hitting made him one of the greatest legends in baseball history. But there were three strikes in Mickey's life that eventually punched him out.

Fame brought Mantle a private life studded with parties and nights on the town. This celebrity lifestyle led him into a 43-year battle with alcohol abuse. Strike one.

The second strike was his "full-bore" attitude, which both fueled his great career and led to its early end. "Mickey never played anything safe. He didn't play his life safe, and he certainly didn't play baseball in a safe fashion. Whatever it took, he played as hard as he could to win the game," says Mickey's former attorney and longtime friend, Roy True. "By the time he left baseball (at age 36), he could not even run, his knees were so bad," says True.

Even though drinking and numerous operations had taken their toll on Mantle's body, he never thought much of it in his glory days. "I was young, and I figured that I was never gonna make it to old. So I was gonna have fun while I could," he said. "If I knew I was going to make it to 50, I would have taken better care of myself."

Mickey's drinking didn't slow down much until the day he checked into the Betty Ford Treatment Center in 1994.

But the damage to Mantle's liver was already done.

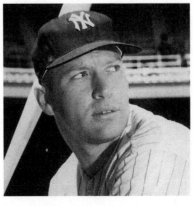

In 1995, he needed an emergency transplant operation for his by-then severely cirrhotic liver. During the surgery to implant the donated liver, the doctors discovered cancer—strike three. "It was referred to in the Baylor Hospital here in Dallas as one of the most aggressive cancers that they had ever seen in any case," True says. Mickey Mantle died in Dallas on August 13, 1995, at age 63.

Within the precious extra weeks that his donor liver bought him, he valiantly told the tragic message of his life—of how his mistakes had hurt him, his family, and his career—warning others of the dangers of drugs and alcohol, in the hope that by using himself as an example, he might affect some lives for the better. He warned others: "Don't drink or do drugs. Your health is the main thing you have, so don't blow it."

By the end of his baseball career, the Mick had won four American League home run titles, the triple crown in 1956, and three American League Most Valuable Player awards. He is still the all-time World Series leader with 18 home runs, 42 runs, 40 RBIs, and 123 total bases. We can only wonder what he could have accomplished had he taken better care of himself.

Aside from learning from his errors, True says that men can perhaps best honor Mantle by helping fulfill his final wish: "If you want to do something great," he said, "be a donor." An organ donor, that is. Overwhelmed by the selfless gift he received, Mantle created the Mickey Mantle Foundation to promote awareness of the need for organ and tissue donation.

To learn more about the plight of the more than 55,000 Americans awaiting organ donations and what you can do about it, write to the Mickey Mantle Foundation, 8080 North Central Expressway, Suite 800, Dallas, TX 75206-1887.

John McSherry

Out at Home Plate

You probably don't recognize his name, but chances are that you remember how he died. Home plate umpire John McSherry called a time-out just seven pitches into the Cincinnati Reds' 1996 season opener. He took a few steps toward the backstop and motioned for help. Then, in a horrifying moment that was broadcast again and again on the evening news, McSherry fell face-first to the ground. When efforts by the team doctors and trainers failed to revive him, the 51-year-old umpire was carried off the field on a stretcher and rushed to a nearby hospital. He was pronounced dead about an hour later. A massive heart attack had taken a man who was all heart.

"Everybody, I mean everybody, loved John McSherry," National League umpire Paul Runge told reporters. "There is good and bad in every profession, and John was the best."

McSherry cared whether he made the right call and wasn't afraid to admit to a bad call. "He's one of the few umpires who will tell you, 'I missed one,' " Reds first baseman Hal Morris said at the time.

But McSherry was more than an umpire; he also was a fan. "All the players loved John McSherry," Chicago Cubs third-base coach Tony Muser told reporters. "When a player had a good game, the next day he'd tell him about it."

Known among the players and umpires as Big John, McSherry was one of the heaviest major league umpires at a time when nearly one in three umpires were over-weight. At almost 400 pounds, McSherry had been pulled from four games in the years prior to his death for dizziness and heat exhaustion. He also had an ab-normal heartbeat and planned to see a doctor the day after he died to begin treatment for the condition. "A lot of us thought

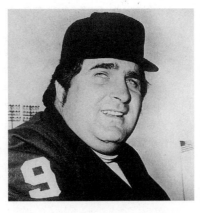

he would retire after last season," Houston Astros outfielder John Cangelosi said at the time. "There were games where he would have diffi-culty breathing and get winded and tired."

"He lived and died an umpire," says Mc-Sherry's best friend and fellow umpire Eric Gregg, who took a leave of absence from um-piring to lose weight just weeks after McSherry's death. "I weighed close to 400 pounds and had an abnormal heartbeat just like Big John did, and I also had high blood pressure. I realized that it could have been me out on the field, and I decided that I better do something about it."

In 18 months, Gregg (who is in his mid-forties) lost 105 pounds, allowing him to cut his heart and blood pressure medication in half. He now walks five to eight miles at least five times a week and swims an hour every day. Gone are the days when he and McSherry would throw down a couple of beers, a prime rib end cut, and a baked potato after a game. Gregg no longer skips breakfast, and at lunch forgoes Philly cheese steaks and burgers for a salad, a slice of bread with tuna, and diet soda.

Gregg, who has dieted before but always gained the weight back, says that this time it's more than a diet—it's a lifestyle change. He even has a strategy to deal with temptations. He wears a silver bracelet inscribed with the words "Big John" on it. "Every time I pick up something that I shouldn't be having and try to put it in my mouth, I look at the bracelet, and it's like Big John is saying, 'You shouldn't have that.' "

Gregg says that McSherry, who was his in-structor at umpire school in 1971, "was like a father figure to me. He gave me a lot of ad-vice." Of all the lessons McSh-erry taught Gregg, probably the most important is that life can end as quickly as a fastball crosses the plate. And at 105 pounds lighter, Gregg intends to be calling those balls and strikes for a long time to come.

Steve Prefontaine

Racing to the Finish

Seven thousand fans packed the stands at the University of Oregon's Hayward Field on May 29, 1975—not for a rock concert or monster truck rally, but to watch their favorite son run. Steve Prefontaine—24 years old, eyes bright with determination, shaggy hair flopping in the wind—won the race, as he had won every other race over a mile at Hayward Field.

Prefontaine, nicknamed "Pre" early in life, ran fiercely that day, as he did every race. Virtually unbeatable on the track, he had shattered dozens of records and took fourth in the 1972 Olympic 5,000-meter race. But driving home from a post-race victory celebration that night in his MGB, Pre misjudged a curve, drove off the road, and crashed into a rock wall nearby. Pre's car flipped over, crushing him inside.

"I will never again experience a shock like learning that Pre was dead," says Kenny Moore, former Olympic marathoner and *Sports Illustrated* writer in Kailua, Hawaii. "Eugene, Oregon, and the running community were absolutely staggered."

Prefontaine grew up in Coos Bay, Oregon, a gritty coastal town where mild temperatures belie winter storms that bring winds of 100 miles an hour. Fishermen and loggers toil to make ends meet in the rugged landscape.

"Pre grew up in a blue-collar community. You have to prove yourself there or else you're going to get chewed up," says Don Kardong, senior writer for *Runner's World* magazine, president of the Road Runners Club of America, and himself a fourth-place finisher in the 1976 Olympic marathon, who lives in Spokane, Washington. "Pre looked around for a sport. He found success in running and channeled all of his desire to

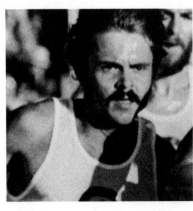

succeed there. Combine that with his great talent and he became spectacular."

Bill Bowerman, former head coach of the University of Oregon's track team in Eugene, described Prefontaine as "a very fierce competitor—the best runner in America. When he came to college, he was the best high school miler in the United States. Pre was like a lot of youngsters: He thought he knew the answers before he heard the questions. He was confident almost to the point of being too much a showman. But I don't think you should act like a pussycat if you're a tiger."

Often, Pre would predict the outcome of his own races, cockily telling a friend or reporter whom he was going to pass and when. "Then, when he sprinted past the favorite, he'd wave," Bowerman says. "That meant the race was over." With his talent and charisma, Pre fast became a fan favorite. When he raced, the stands filled with people chanting, "Go Pre." "He loved to hear the crowd," Bowerman says. "I think it was a great lift for him."

Although brash and bold, Pre cared deeply about his family, friends, competitors, and the sport of running.

"Pre's love of the crowd, of *his* people, was a two-way street," Moore says. "He worked with kids, and he started a running club for prisoners. He gloried in being an outspoken member of his community and wanting to make it better."

More than 20 years after his death, the exact cause of Pre's crash is still unknown. Perhaps the night of his accident, alcohol impaired his driving; perhaps he swerved to avoid an oncoming car; perhaps he drifted off to sleep for just a second.

Pre's family and friends still wonder: If only he had less to drink, if only he had left the party sooner, if only he had worn his seat belt, would he still be alive?

Index